OXFORD MEDICAL PUBLICATIONS

Psychopharmacology and sexual disorders

BRITISH ASSOCIATION FOR PSYCHOPHARMACOLOGY MONOGRAPHS

Psychopharmacology and sexual disorders

BRITISH ASSOCIATION
FOR PSYCHOPHARMACOLOGY
MONOGRAPH
No. 4

EDITED BY
DAVID WHEATLEY

*Head, Psychopharmacology Research
Group, Twickenham*

OXFORD NEW YORK TOKYO
OXFORD UNIVERSITY PRESS
1983

Oxford University Press, Walton Street, Oxford OX2 6DP

London Glasgow New York Toronto
Delhi Bombay Calcutta Madras Karachi
Kuala Lumpur Singapore Hong Kong Tokyo
Nairobi Dar es Salaam Cape Town
Melbourne Auckland

and associates in
Beirut Berlin Ibadan Mexico City Nicosia

OXFORD is a trade mark of Oxford University Press

British Library Cataloguing in Publication Data
Psychopharmacology and sexual disorders. –
(British Association for Psychopharmacology
monographs; no. 4). – (Oxford medical publications)
1. Sexual disorders – Chemo therapy
I. Wheatley, David, 1919-   II. Series
616.6'9061   RC556
ISBN 0-19-261415-0

Library of Congress Cataloging in Publication Data
Main entry under title:
Psychopharmacology and sexual disorders.
(A British Association for Psychopharmacology
monograph; no. 4)
Proceedings of the annual summer meeting of the
British Association for Psychopharmacology, 1982,
at the Royal Society.
Includes bibliographical references and index.
1. Sexual disorders – Congresses.   2. Psychosexual
disorders – Congresses.   3. Psychopharmacology –
Congresses.   I. Wheatley, David, 1919-
II. British Association for Psychopharmacology.
III. Series.
RC556.P747 1983   616.6'9061   83-12147
ISBN 0-19-261415-0

Set by Hope Services, Abingdon
Printed and bound in Great Britain by
William Clowes Limited, Beccles and London

Preface

London was the venue for the annual summer meeting of the British Association for Psychopharmacology (BAP) in 1982, the meeting being held jointly with the Biological Psychiatry Section of the Royal College of Psychiatrists. The principal contribution from the BAP to the meeting was a symposium on 'Psychopharmacology and Sexual Disorders' and it is on this symposium that the present volume is based. However, the speakers have expanded their papers and the topic has been more comprehensively covered by including a number of additional contributors.

The meeting was held at the Royal Society, overlooking the Mall, under the benevolent gaze of Charles II, the Royal founder and first Patron of the Royal Society, whose portrait hangs behind the Chairman's seat. What thoughts, per-chance, might have passed through the mind of the merry monarch could he have overheard the serious debate that was taking place on one of his favourite subjects. Perplexed indeed he might have been to learn of the taboos and myths that have been built up about that most normal human function of all, sexual activity. In his day and age, the physical diseases resulting from the pursuit of sexual pleasure might have seemed a terrible retribution from above, but it is doubtful whether fear of this in any way inhibited the natural fulfilment of nature's urges.

Indeed, the Victorian era, with its system of double-standards in so many areas of social life, must be blamed for many of the psychiatric and psychologi-cal sequelae that we observe today, as a result of the inhibitions and guilt feelings imposed upon the present generation by their forebears. Many of the problems that constitute disorders of sexual functioning stem from such a deep-rooted psychological background, and it is therefore appropriate to consider the role that psychopharmacology has to play, in attempting to rectify the errors of the past in this area. However, in assessing the role of psychopharmacology in the treatment of sexual disorders, this must be viewed against the background of basic research into the cerebral processes involved in the sexual act, and against the effectiveness of other forms of treatment, such as psychotherapy and treatment with non-psychotropic drugs.

The volume is divided into three sections entitled respectively: Sex in the Laboratory, Sex in the Community, and Sex and Drugs. The first part is con-cerned with basic research into the mechanisms of the normal sexual functions and derangements that may occur when dysfunction supervenes. Next, Sex in the Community is concerned with the psychiatric and psychological influences that affect sexuality and some of the external factors, such as age and alcohol for example, that may influence these. In the final section, drugs that may influence sexual function are considered in depth, in relation to the central mechanisms involved and the manner in which they may act on sexual functioning, be this by way of impairment, restoration to normal or even enhancement.

The opening chapter of Sex in the Laboratory is contributed by Everitt and Hansen and describes the interactions between catecholamines and hypothalamic mechanisms, in relation to the control of sexual behaviour. These data have been gathered from the results of experiments in male and female rats, and suggest that the noradrenaline system may be important in the control of mounting behaviour and even ejaculation in the male, and the level of receptivity in the female.

The role that neurotransmitters may play in sexual functioning is expanded by Gessa of Sardinia in the next chapter, who specifically considers premature ejaculation in rats. Not only can this condition be induced experimentally, but may occur spontaneously in some less fortunate members of the rat community. Rather than feeling insulted that, in this respect at least, man is no better than rat, consolation may be found in the reflection that man, at least, is potentially capable of solving such problems. The fact that dopamine agonists can produce premature ejaculation in rats with ease, leads to the inescapable conclusion that the dopaminergic system must be intimately involved in control of sexual mechanisms. The inference for clinical psychopharmacology is that dopamine receptor blockers might provide a logical form of treatment for this apparently trivial but nevertheless highly distressing condition, with its inevitable psychological sequelae.

The role of neurones in sexual activity is considered further in Chapter 3 by Tucker and File, who describe the results of their experiments in rats in relation to serotonin mechanisms. It would seem well established that male patterns of sexual behaviour are enhanced in both sexes as a result of lowering brain 5-hydroxytryptamine (5-HT). The authors speculate as to the relevance of their results in the rat in relation to man, but the increased sexual performance resulting from association between adolescent male rats and mature females (the older woman effect), would seem to suggest a direct parallel to the human situation.

The effects of psychotropic drugs in any malfunction of the psyche or neuro-psyche is intimately related to the endocrine system and in particular the pituitary. Recent developments in the identification of specific receptors for opiods and benzodiazepines in the brain, provide striking proof of this association, as does the development of the dexamethasone-suppression test for the differential diagnosis of depression.

In Chapter 4, Hans Kopera of Austria considers the relationships between hormones affecting sexual behaviour and the brain, emphasizing that the results of animal experiments and experiences in man certainly indicate the brain to be one of their target organs. The identification of specific receptors for oestrogens and progestins provides additional evidence for this.

In the final chapter of this section, Ismet Karacan and his colleagues from Houston, turn their attention to the human species in the laboratory setting.

Understanding of the basic neuro-psychiatric mechanisms that take place in the preamble to copulation and in the act itself, have been enormously advanced by the pioneering studies of Masters and Johnson. However, nature provides a much more subtle approach to observation of the mechanics of sex in the male, namely the changes that occur in penile status during that phase of sleep characterized by rapid eye movements (REM). This has been put to good use by Karacan and his colleagues, in the precise measurement of the mechanics involved in nocturnal penile tumescence (NPT), and the new approach that this offers to the diagnosis and treatment of impotence in the male. How sad indeed that nature does not provide a similar paradigm for the female.

Leaving the laboratory, the theme of the book is now continued in relation to the community of man. Three of the contributors to this section of the book come from the USA, emphasizing the far greater importance that is placed on the understanding of both normal and abnormal sexual patterns in that country, as compared to the somewhat hidebound attitudes that have prevailed in the United Kingdom. Alex Comfort from Los Angeles discusses the anxieties that can and so often do develop from misunderstandings concerning normal sexual function. Psychotropic drugs can also be involved in an adverse manner and it is important to understand the effects of such drugs on sexual functions, lest they enhance the symptoms for the relief of which they were prescribed in the first place. It may be that the present generation of psychotropic drugs has only a minor role to play in this area, but clinicians should not overlook the basic relevance of their modes of action, particularly in relation to newer compounds that may be developed in the future.

Domeena Renshaw of Chicago considers the problems that arise in relation to waning sexual function due to advancing age, the effects of illnesses, and the mechanical interference of physical disabilities. In years gone by, it would have been considered to be totally inappropriate that an elderly couple should even want the affinity of a sexual relationship, albeit unconsummated; whilst the concept of a cripple attempting to indulge his or her natural instincts would have been viewed with revulsion. Small wonder that sexual problems play such an important part in the multitude of individuals whose life is already marred by their physical ailments and how true is her recurring theme: 'If you don't use it, you'll lose it'.

Patricia Gillan in her chapter considers a vital aspect of sex counselling, perhaps the most effective method for treating most sexual disorders and against the background of which, the contribution from psychopharmacology must be judged. She is concerned with aspects of communication, not only between man and his consort or woman and her consort, but also between therapist and patient. Her discourse is refreshing in that she has achieved a total elimination of all inhibitions in the style of her narrative. It is perhaps symptomatic of the penultimate generation that the editor of this volume himself was occasionally tempted to alter her phraseology. More shame to him that it should be so.

Karacan and Moore who provide the final chapter to this section, consider one of the most important social influences on the sexual pattern of peoples' lives, namely that of alcohol. Alcohol, that ambivalent servant of man, that can so inflame sexual desire as to overcome the inhibitions that inhibit and yet may also completely suppress that which is desired, is indeed man's 'oldest tranquillizer'. No wonder then that it exerts a finely tuned psychotropic influence in relation to sexual disorders, depending on the mode of administration and the circumstances of it's consumption.

As Alan and Elizabeth Riley point out in the opening chapter of the section on Sex and Drugs, as many as 30 per cent of patients presenting with sexual difficulties are found to have an organic abnormality, thus indicating possibilities for a pharmacological approach to treatment. They have studied drugs that influence the cholinergic and adrenergic systems in human volunteers with some fascinating results. To quote but two examples, they used a number of ingenious methods to assess the quality of orgasm in females in response to cholinergic stimulation, and the effects of adrenergic stimulation on delayed ejaculation and orgasm in the male. But the chapter must be read in full to appreciate the fascinating pharmacological possibilities that may lie ahead in consequence of studies such as these.

These putative therapeutic uses of drugs are counter-balanced by the adverse effects on sexual function of psychotropic drugs that may be prescribed for other reasons. This subject is considered by John Rees of Manchester in Chapter 11, but the latter must be seen in the context of the aetiology of sexual disorders since, for example, prescribed drugs contribute to less than 5 per cent of all the organic causes of impotence, psychogenic factors being infinitely more important. Sexual side-effects of prescribed drugs, both psychotropic and other, are often given scant attention in manufacturers literature; patients themselves may be hesitant to complain of them, and may not appreciate that they are due to the drugs prescribed. The attitude of many physicians does not help either, since adverse effects on sexual functioning are so often dismissed as totally unimportant in relation to the treatment being prescribed, as for example in hypertension. However, it must be recalled that so often long-term drug treatment is a 'life sentence' and that some patients might prefer a reduced life expectancy, in return for a full return to sexual enjoyment over the intervening years. More importantly, consideration should be given to alternative drugs or forms of therapy that can be considered, and that do not interfere with sexual functions.

Aphrodisiacs — do they really exist? Robert Greenblatt and his colleagues from Georgia, USA, have appropriately added the rider 'in legend and in fact' to the title of their chapter. Alcohol, oysters, cantharides, yohimbine, and pornography amongst many others, are all attributed to stimulate or revive sexual prowess, but, as the authors point out, the only true aphrodisiac is testosterone. Other methods may well act through the power of suggestion and, of course, this should not be ignored. In the context of the title of this volume, it is reassuring to read in the conclusion to their chapter that Greenblatt and his colleagues comment: 'in a measure testosterone is a psychotropic drug'.

The final chapter of the volume is concerned with a different aspect of the subject, namely drug control of excessive sexual urges in the male. Of a number of psychotropic drugs that have been used for this purpose, the most promising are the anti-androgens but the problem of patient compliance still remains, as Christopher Mugglestone, the author of the chapter, points out. Nevertheless, he does not consider that the solution lies in the discovery of either a more specific anti-androgen or even in the development of a long-acting injectible preparation to overcome problems of compliance, but rather in further elucidation of the pathogenesis of the condition. And indeed this is a fitting epitaph to this section, emphasizing as it does that although there are a variety of drugs both psychotropic and other that are widely prescribed to treat sexual disorders, very little is really known about the underlying pathogenesis or the specificity of indications for individual drug therapies.

The ethics of artificially enhancing libido and the perception of sexual pleasure, would have been considered dubious indeed in days gone by. But now, provided that they are harmless or relatively harmless, the prescribing of 'pleasure drugs' must be seriously considered by the physician, not only in matters sexual but in the chemical regulation of mood as well. Reference has already been made in the previous volume in this series (Wheatley, D. 1982. Editorial. *Psychopharmacology of old age*. OUP, Oxford), to the importance of ensuring sleep in the elderly when this is psychologically desirable although physiologically unnecessary. Similar arguments apply to the maintenance and improvement of sexual satisfaction when this is possible, particularly when dysfunction supervenes as the result of increasing age, illness, or other reasons, as outlined in some of the chapters of this book.

The lack of specific psychotropic or other drugs to achieve these objectives underlines an important gap in the practice of psychiatry, the speciality that is so intimately concerned with the mental and emotional well-being of the patient. Whilst awaiting such a therapeutic advance, some thought might be given to the psychological overlay that is so often present in sexual disorders. Surely some ingenuous drug manufacturer could concoct a simple harmless formulation, possibly with psychotropic ingredients, that could be prescribed to treat psychogenic sexual abnormalities? The need for such a preparation is underlined by the recent withdrawal from the British market of such a combination which, although it was probably relatively inert, nevertheless had many therapeutic successes attributed to it. In this context also, since we not only condone the use of other 'pleasure drugs' such as alcohol, nicotine, and caffeine, it might now be considered laudable also to investigate the possibilities for producing a safe and effective aphrodisiac. Mankind would be much the better for its discovery.

Twickenham　　　　　　　　　　　　　　　　　　　　　　　　D.W.
January 1983

Contents

Contributors

C. ASLAN,
Department of Psychiatry,
Baylor College of Medicine,
Houston

J. CHADDHA,
Department of Endocrinology,
Medical College of Georgia,
Augusta

A. COMFORT,
Neurophychiatric Institute,
UCLA,
Los Angeles

B. J. EVERITT,
Department of Anatomy,
University of Cambridge

S. E. FILE,
Department of Pharmacology,
The School of Pharmacy,
London

G. L. GESSA,
Institute of Pharmacology,
University of Cagliari

P. GILLAN,
Institute of Psychiatry and Maudsley Hospital,
London

R. B. GREENBLATT,
Department of Endocrinology,
Medical School of Georgia,
Augusta

S. HANSEN,
Department of Psychology,
University of Goteborg

I. KARACAN,
Sleep Disorders and Research Center,
Baylor College of Medicine,
Houston

H. KOPERA,
Department of Experimental and Clinical Psychology,
Karl-Franzens-Universität,
Graz

C. A. MOORE,
Department of Psychiatry,
Baylor College of Medicine,
Houston

C. J. MUGGLESTONE,
Medical/Scientific Division,
Brocades Ltd.,
West Byfleet

L. NAPOLI-FARRIS,
Institute of Pharmacology,
University of Cagliari

J. M. H. REES,
Department of Pharmacology,
Materia Medica and Therapeutics,
University of Manchester Medical School

D. C. RENSHAW,
Department of Psychiatry and Sexual Dysfunction Clinic,
Loyola University,
Chicago

A. J. RILEY,
Touchwood House,
Wendens Ambo,
Saffron Walden

E. J. RILEY,
Touchwood House,
Wendesn Ambo,
Saffron Walden

C. SAMARAS,
Department of Endocrinology,
Medical College of Georgia,
Augusta

J. C. TUCKER,
Department of Pharmacology,
The School of Pharmacy,
London

C. VERHEUGEN,
Department of Endocrinology,
Medical College of Georgia,
Augusta

R. L. WILLIAMS,
Department of Psychiatry,
Baylor College of Medicine,
Houston

Sex in the laboratory

1

Catecholamines and hypothalamic mechanisms

B. J. EVERITT AND S. HANSEN

INTRODUCTION

THE STUDY of the physiological basis of motivated behaviour has, over the years, been undertaken within several theoretical frameworks. In one early formulation (Stellar 1954) the importance of specific and multiple hypothalamic drive 'centres', acted upon by various internal signals according to the bodily state of the organism, was regarded as the key mechanism underlying motivation. This view was based primarily on the impressive changes in motivated behaviour observed after lesions and stimulations of the hypothalamus. An alternative model (Hebb 1955) held that motivated behaviour emerged out of the need to maintain an optimal level of arousal, set out of balance by various internal deficit states and external cues. Here, the brain stem reticular formation and its long-recognized role in arousal mechanisms, replaced the drives of the hypothalamus as the primary neural substrate for motivation (Mogenson and Phillips 1976).

Both formulations continue to influence behavioural research in such a way that contemporary neurobiological analysis of motivation is often directed towards finding ways in which to link the two. For instance, does the neural circuitry underlying goal-directed behaviours involve some interaction between relatively specific 'hypothalamic drive systems' and brain stem mechanisms mediating more generalized behavioural functions (e.g. arousal or reward)? According to this view, certain patterns of hypothalamic activity might promote the development of particular arousal states, or increase the rewarding properties of certain sensory inputs.

In this chapter we will discuss, within the general framework outlined above, the ways in which sex hormones, acting primarily in the hypothalamus, and catecholaminergic (CA) neurones, forming part of the brain stem reticular formation (Moore 1980), might interact in the control of sexual behaviour.

ROLE OF THE HYPOTHALAMUS

That the hypothalamus is a critical component in the neural circuitry mediating sexual behaviour has been established beyond doubt. Recent work emphasizes the importance of the ventromedial nucleus (VMN) and the medial preoptic area (MPOA), in the regulation of feminine and masculine patterns of sexual behaviour, respectively.

This is for several reasons. Firstly, steroid hormones known to regulate patterns of mating behaviour are actively taken up and retained by a great number of VMN and MPOA neurones, many of which have been demonstrated to possess specialized receptors for androgens, oestrogens, and progestagens, as well as the aromatase enzymes which are so important in some species to produce the behaviourally active metabolite of testosterone, oestradiol (see review by McEwen, Davis, Parsons, and Pfaff, 1979). Secondly, while the VMN and MPOA share with many other structures of the brain and spinal cord the ability to concentrate sex hormones, studies involving the implantation of these hormones emphasize the importance of these two hypothalamic populations of steroid-sensitive neurones, in the control of sexual behaviour.

Hormone implantation

Minute steroid pellets located in the rostral hypothalamus are considerably more effective than implants in other sites in the brain, to reactivate mounting behaviour in castrated male rats (Davidson 1966). Thus, 70 per cent of a group of castrated rats bearing oestradiol implants in the MPOA region showed the ejaculatory pattern in contrast to only 10 per cent of males implanted with similar hormone pellets in the posterior hypothalamus (Christensen and Clemens 1974). In ovariectomized rats, recent evidence suggests that when the proper precautions are taken to minimize the spread of hormone release by the steroid pellet, the VMN stands out as being uniquely sensitive to the receptivity-inducing actions of oestradiol (Davis, McEwen, and Pfaff 1979; Rubin and Barfield 1980).

There is also evidence to suggest that progesterone, which normally times and intensifies the mating behaviour of oestrogen-primed rats (Hansen and Sodersten 1979), also acts in the ventromedial hypothalamus (Rubin and Barfield 1981). Finally, it is well known that certain hypothalamic lesions permanently abolish sexual behaviour, without necessarily impairing the secretion of steroid hormones from the gonads. Electrolytic lesions of the VMN, especially its lateral portion, are associated with poor lordosis performance in rodents; according to Pfaff and Sakuma (1979) sexual receptivity declines gradually over a 48 h long period following lesioning, with partial recovery occurring over the next 2 weeks. In male rats, lesions situated in the MPOA, and typically encompassing also the adjacent anterior hypothalamic area, permanently abolish copulatory behaviour. Indeed, as assessed by the lesioning approach at least, the functional integrity of the MPOA seems to be a necessary prerequisite for the complete mating pattern in all vertebrates studied to date (which include several amphibian, avian, and mammalian species). Perhaps the most noteworthy finding here is the reduction and, in some cases, even complete elimination of mounting activity in male rhesus monkeys bearing MPOA lesions (Slimp, Hart, and Goy 1978).

In an attempt to characterize in more detail the nature of the hypothalamic damage so effective in reducing male copulatory patterns throughout the phylogenetic scale, Hansen, Köhler, Goldstein, and Steinbusch (1982a) compared the behavioural consequences of MPOA electrocoagulations with microinjection of ibotenic acid, an axon- and terminal-sparing neurotoxic agent which appears to degenerate only nerve cell bodies in the exposed region (Schwarcz, Hökfelt, Fuxe, Jonsson, Goldstein, and Terenius 1979). It was found that the selective degeneration of neuronal perikarya was sufficient to completely abolish mounting activity of male rats, and it is likely, therefore, that the nerve cell bodies of the MPOA, and their neuronal projections, constitute the critical component for sexual behaviour within this part of the brain.

Catecholaminergic neurones

Having discussed so far the importance of hormone-sensitive hypothalamic mechanisms in the control of sexual behaviour, let us now examine the possibility that CA neurones of the brain stem are of significance in this neuro-endocrine system. Studies employing sensitive tract-tracing methods have amply confirmed Nauta's concept of a 'limbic midbrain', and thus the possibility that steroid-responsive basal forebrain structures might influence the activity of CA neurones originating in, or coursing through, the midbrain (Nauta and Haymaker 1969). For example, recent autoradiographic evidence (summarized by Swanson and Mogenson 1981) shows that the MPOA, by virtue of its extensive neuronal projections, is in a position to influence not only the autonomic nervous system (by way of its projections to several hypothalamic nuclei which in turn send axons to preganglionic autonomic cell groups) and the secretions of the pituitary gland (via projections to the median eminence), but probably also the activity of catecholamine neurones. The latter may be influenced especially by way of MPOA efferents to the ventral tegmental area, the reticular formation of the midbrain, and the lateral hypothalamus/medial forebrain bundle (LH/MFB) system. In silver impregnation studies of brains bearing MPOA lesions (similar in size to those abolishing sex behaviour in the rat), the terminal degeneration in the LH/MFB is particularly impressive (Hansen, unpublished results). This points to the distinct possibility that hormone-sensitive preoptic neurones may modulate the activity of ascending dopaminergic (DA) and noradrenergic (NA) fibre tracts, within the LH/MFB.

As we have discussed, NA and DA neurones ascending from the brain stem and distributed widely over the neuraxis, form parts of neural systems very different to the steroid-sensitive systems present in the hypothalamus and limbic system which are critically linked to the control of sexual behaviour. What, then, is the evidence for the involvement of CA-dependent processes in the control of sexual behaviour? Can we define the nature of these processes and their relationship to the hormone-dependent mechanisms described above? It should be emphasized at the outset that NA and DA neurones do not subserve functions *specific* to the control of sexual behaviour, it being well known that manipulation of CA transmission alters a wide variety of goal-directed activities. Our problem then, is to specify the context in which CA neurone activity is a determinant of sexual responses (Everitt 1978; Meyerson and Malmnäs 1978; Robbins and Everitt 1982).

Early on, the demonstration by Malmnäs (1973) that blocking catecholamine synthesis with the CA synthesis inhibitor, α-methyl-p-tyrosine, markedly reduced masculine sexual behaviour (along with most other goal-directed behaviours), pointed to a fundamental role of the CAs in the expression of sexual behaviour. According to Caggiula, Shaw, Antelman, and Edwards (1976), who studied male rats injected intracerebroventricularly with 6 hydroxydopamine (6-OHDA) to degenerate central CA neurones, this role may at least partly consist of maintaining proper responsiveness to stimuli eliciting approach and mounting in the male, or the proceptive behaviour of an oestrous female.

Pharmacological approaches

Attempts by pharmacological means to identify which of the two major CA systems mediates the effects of these drug treatments have mostly pointed to the DA pathways. Whilst several DA receptor blockers potently reduce the mounting behaviour of male rats (Baum and Starr 1980), blocking of adrenergic α- or β-receptors seems to leave sexual behaviour unaffected (Malmnäs 1973). Administration of the DA receptor agonist, apomorphine, results in facilitation of several aspects of the mating pattern, such that rats ejaculate with a shorter latency and after fewer intromissions (Paglietti, Pellegrini-Quarantotti, Merev, and Gessa 1978), although in independent studies in our laboratories this effect has proved to be very variable (unpublished data).

In the female, like the male, the use of drugs which modulate NA transmission has resulted in a very confused picture so far as revealing NA mechanisms in the organization of sexual responses is concerned (see Everitt, Fuxe, Hokfelt, and Jonsson 1976). However, DA receptor agonist and antagonist drugs have effects on the sexual behaviour of female rodents, which both emphasize similarities to studies on the male, and also great differences which are related to the *nature* of female sexual responses. Thus, drugs which decrease DA transmission are associated with a profound increase in the display of lordosis, which might be interpreted as an increase in receptivity (Everitt, Fuxe, and Hokfelt 1974). However, the same drug treatment also markedly decreases the display of proceptive behaviours, which may readily be interpreted as reduced sexual motivation; effects comparable to those seen in the male (Caggiula, Antelman, Chiodo, and Lineberry 1979a; Caggiula, Hernden, Scanlon, Greenstone, Bradshaw, and Sharp 1979b; Robbins and Everitt 1982). The explanation for this apparent paradox resides in the nature of the female's behavioural repertoire. Proceptivity is a highly active pattern of behaviour while receptive responses require immobility. The latter is consistent with, indeed enhanced by, DA blockade, but the same treatment prevents the expression of active motor patterns, such as proceptivity. Clearly, the expression of these hormone-dependent behaviours is much affected by manipulation of the DA system. It is important to resolve the nature of this influence of DA mechanisms, in both male and female, particularly with regard to motor response patterns which typify sexual behaviour in each sex.

CATECHOLAMINE PATHWAYS

Pharmacological data such as these would seem to encourage a careful exploration of the contributions of individual CA pathways in different components of sexual behaviour. The necessary prerequisites for this sort of analysis, i.e. information as to the distribution in the CNS of the DA and NA pathways, combined with relatively specific tools (e.g. 6-OHDA) with which to manipulate

1978). As yet, however, relatively few studies of this kind seem to have been conducted, though substantial behavioural effects have been seen to follow non-selective lesions in areas known to be abundant in catecholamine neurones.

Studies in male rats

Electrocoagulations situated in the LH/MFB system reduce markedly the copulatory activity of male rats (Hitt, Hendricks, Ginsberg, and Lewis 1970) and the possibility remains that these effects are, to a significant extent, due to damage to ascending CA neurones (e.g. the nigrostriatal DA axons) running in the MFB. This interpretation receives some support from the finding that restricted axon-sparing lesions, induced by ibotenic acid-infusions in the LH/ MFB, at a site where electrocoagulations are disruptive (Hitt *et al.* 1970), do not affect sexual behaviour (Hansen, Köhler, Goldstein, and Steinbusch 1982*a*), but effects of lesions encompassing the entire projection field of MPOA neurones in the LH/MFB have yet to be fully explored. A second example of a presumed CA involvement in copulatory behaviour concerns a report by Barfield, Wilson, and McDonald (1975) showing that lesions of the ventral tegmental area which, among other things, contains the A10 cluster giving rise to the DA innervation of the ventral striatum and prefrontal cortex (Lindvall and Bjorklund 1978). These facilitated the sexual behaviour of male rats, a conspicuous decrease in the post-ejaculatory refractory period being the most prominent effect.

It would certainly be interesting to know the consequences of more selective manipulations of this region in the brain, although in preliminary experiments it has not proved possible to reproduce the behavioural effects of VTA lesions by 6-OHDA infusions in the prefrontal cortex (S. Hansen, unpublished observations) or into the nucleus accumbens (Fineberg and Everitt, unpublished observations) both of which are major terminal areas of the A10 DA cell group. In the latter experiment, accumbens DA levels 80 per cent lower than in controls were associated with *prolonged* latencies to ejaculate, in the two weeks following the lesion. There was no effect on the post-ejaculatory refractory period and the most conspicuous change in the rats' interactions with females was a prolonged latency to initiate investigation and mounting. The rapid recovery of function following these terminal lesions made long-term analysis of the altered behaviour difficult, and the importance of ventral striatal mechanisms in sexual behaviour remains to be determined.

Decreased post-ejaculatory refractoriness was also noted by Clark, Caggiula, McConnell, and Antelman (1975) following lesions in the dorsal midbrain and, since they were situated in the region of the dorsal NA bundle and caused major depletions in telencephalic NA content, it was suggested that the inhibition of sexual activity which occurs after ejaculation requires activity in this system of central NA neurones. In a subsequent study, however, Clark (1980) failed to reproduce the effect of the non-specific lesions by local 6-OHDA infusions in the same site. Hansen, Köhler, and Ross (1982*b*) concluded on the basis of studies employing ibotenic acid and DSP4, that the integrity of a non-adrenergic fibre system (as yet unidentified) running in the dorsal tegmental bundle, may be necessary for post-ejaculatory refractoriness of normal duration. It was additionally found that males subjected to central NA depletion by DSP4, which degenerates NA nerve terminal projections derived primarily from the locus coeruleus (Jonsson 1980), were consistently slower than controls to ejaculate and exhibited *prolonged* refractory periods (Hansen *et al*. 1982*b*). The latter effect is likely to be due to damage to descending NA projections because it has recently been found (Hansen and Ross 1982) that 6-OHDA infusions into the spinal subarachnoid space, reducing the synaptosomal uptake of tritiated NA in spinal cord by more than 50 per cent whilst leaving hippocampal uptake unaffected, similarly increased the duration of the post-ejaculatory refractory period. Spinal NA denervation also appeared to render the male rats more sensitive to hormone deprivation, since they ceased to copulate sooner after castration than controls (Hansen and Ross 1982).

In an independent study (Taylor and Everitt, unpublished observations, 1982), infusions of 6-OHDA into descending NA axons in the cervical spinal cord also· resulted in prolonged latencies to ejaculate. This appeared to be a consequence of disturbed temporal patterning of mounts and intromissions. Thus, prolonged latencies to the first mount, prolonged inter-mount intervals, and fewer intromissions followed these injections (which were associated with 90 per cent depletions of NA at all levels of the cord, but no change in hypothalamus or cerebral cortex). Some animals failed to ejaculate during the first post-operative 30-min test, but only two (of 12) persisted in not ejaculating. In four rats, behavioural signs of ejaculation were observed, but spermatozoa could not be detected in post-coital vaginal smears. This result of spinal NA depletion on ejaculation requires confirmation. Again, the remarkable functional recovery which occurred 2–3 weeks after the lesion made detailed analysis of these effects difficult to achieve. However, these preliminary data would seem to suggest that spinal NA projections may be important in modulating spinal events associated with the patterning of mounts and, perhaps, ejaculation. Whether these changes reflect the influence of NA in the dorsal horn (and sensory events), the ventral horn (and motor outflow), or the intermediolateral cell column (both sympathetic and parasympathetic outflow to the genitalia), has not been determined.

Studies in female rats

In females, intracerebral manipulation of DA neurones has profound effects on sexual behaviour. Infusions of 6-OHDA intracerebroventricularly, such that forebrain DA levels are much reduced, were seen to mirror the effects of systemically administered DA antagonists (Caggiula *et al*. 1979*b*). Females so-treated displayed enhanced levels of receptivity but reduced levels of proceptivity. The same workers went on to demonstrate that cervical probing, which induces lordosis, and tail pinch, an activating stimulus, have reciprocal effects on the firing of DA neurones in the substantia nigra (Chiodo, Caggiula, Antelman, and Lineberry 1979). More specific lesions to DA neurones have confirmed this general picture and suggest that active, proceptive behaviours are associated with an activated DA system, while the immobile lordosis posture induced by tactile contact with the male, is associated with decreased DA activity. Thus, injection of 6-OHDA into the VTA of oestadiol-treated female rats, results in the enhanced display of lordosis but no effect on proceptivity (Alton, Wright, and Everitt 1979; Robbins and Everitt 1982). Addition of progesterone, which induces high levels of proceptivity and receptivity in controls, has no additional effect on the high levels of receptivity in VTA-lesioned females, but fails also to induce maximal levels of proceptivity (Alton *et al.* 1979; Parsons, Stanfield, Hansen, and Everitt 1981). Neurochemically, these lesions were associated with significant DA loss in the nucleus accumbens and also the anterior caudate nucleus. Direct injection of 6-OHDA into the nucleus accumbens itself resulted in a behavioural picture rather similar to VTA dopamine lesions (Parsons *et al.* 1981; Robbins and Everitt 1982). Females so-lesioned showed enhanced frequencies and duration of lordotic responses but reduced amounts of proceptivity, when treated with oestradiol and progesterone.

INTERPRETING THE DATA

One interpretation of these data is that consummatory responses are subject to less interruption than usual following lesions of ventral striatal DA, and hence the prolonged lordotic postures following mounting attempts, while the ancillary effects of motivational excitement or activation are reduced, with resultant lower levels of proceptivity. Such a view of the data is consistent with the effects of similar lesions on food- and water-motivated behaviour (Robbins and Everitt 1982). We mention this because it is important to emphasize again that DA neurones, together with other monoaminergic neural systems, have no exclusive role in a single behaviour, but a more general effect on the expression of all goal-directed behaviours. The challenge in the context of sexual behaviour is to determine how the unique, hormone-dependent control mechanisms interact, if they do, with the ubiquitous DA system, to activate the motor patterns of sexual response. We return to this later.

Noradrenergic lesions

Selective lesions of the lateral tegmental NA neurones in the ventral noradrenergic bundle (VNAB), also result in a dissociation of proceptive and receptive behaviours. Females treated with oestradiol and progesterone still display high levels of proceptivity after VNAB lesions, but the capacity to display lordosis is severely impaired (Hansen, Stanfield, and Everitt 1980, 1981). This dissociation also occurs in females bearing their ovaries who show regular 4-day cycles of proceptivity but not receptivity (Hansen *et al.* 1981). This is particularly interesting because it highlights the nature of the stimuli which elicit sexual responses in the female. Clearly, olfactory, visual, and auditory cues emanating from the male, which so specifically induce proceptive responses in the female, continue to do so after VNAB lesions. However lordosis, which is uniquely dependent on tactile cues delivered by the male during a mount, is selectively disrupted by VNAB lesions. We have argued (Hansen *et al.* 1981) that lateral tegmental NA neurones are important, therefore, in enabling behavioural responses to tactile cues associated with coitus.

The location of these NA neurones in the brainstem is consistent with the foregoing view (Hansen *et al.* 1981) and it is interesting that many of them are also oestradiol target neurones (Heritage, Grant, and Stumpf 1977), given the relationship to hormone-dependent events in these experiments. The fact that the same VNAB lesions disrupt the induction of pseudopregnancy following cervical stimulation (Hansen *et al.*, 1981), reinforces the view that these NA neurones are important in a somatosensory setting. That this somatosensory function is particularly pertinent in situations which involve cervical stimulation has received recent support from two very different experimental studies; one involving the olfactory block to pregnancy in mice (the 'Bruce Effect', Keverne and de la Riva 1982), the other involving mother–infant bonding in sheep after parturition (Keverne, Poindron, Levy, and Lindsay 1982). In both instances, NA lesions to the olfactory and accessory olfactory bulbs, the innervation of which originates largely in lateral tegmental cell groups (Everitt and Keverne unpublished results), prevents the selective processing of olfactory cues during and after vaginal/cervical stimulation associated with coitus or parturition.

Taken together, the above results emphasize how a pervasive role of a chemically identified system of neurones can be seen to be important in the rather special conditions which determine the occurrence of sexual behaviour. Thus, NA neurones presumably have importance in a wide variety of behavioural, endocrine, or other physiological settings. Defining the precise nature of their importance is, however, dependent on providing the appropriate conditions to reveal it, in a system where many individual elements operate in an integrated way. In the studies of sexual behaviour outlined above we have touched upon steroidal, noradrenergic, and dopaminergic mechanisms, although there are surely many more, yet even now it is not clear whether any of these interact directly with any other. We were, however, intrigued by the apparently opposing effects of NA and DA lesions on sexual responses in females, in view of persistent reports in the literature of interactions between NA and DA neurones (Robbins and Everitt 1982). One site of such an interaction has been suggested to be the midbrain, particularly the VTA, and it is interesting to note that NA infusions here result in decreased proceptive and increased receptive responses (Parsons *et al.* 1981; Robbins and Everitt 1982), i.e. a pattern opposite to VNAB lesions and similar to VTA/accumbens DA lesions. Whether such direct interaction does reflect one means whereby sensory input from the genitalia alters DA neuronal activity remains to be investigated.

CONCLUSIONS

The current literature on CA involvement in sexual behaviour has still but a fragmented and incomplete picture to offer those wishing to know the function of the various CA pathways in this particular category of goal-directed behaviour. Clearly, much more research on these fundamental issues is required before a coherent, and much-needed, picture can emerge. In particular, we have referred above to the problem of defining any direct relationship between hormone-dependent mechanisms in the hypothalamus, and catecholamine neurones in the medulla, pons, and midbrain.

One recent experiment would appear to be pertinent here. Thus, the remains of the neural circuitry underlying sexual behaviour after hypothalamic damage can be made functional again by manipulating central monoamine systems. More specifically, Hansen *et al.* (1982*a*) have found that daily injections of the semi-synthetic ergoline, lisuride, which interacts with DA and 5-HT receptors (Horowski and Dorow 1981), temporarily restored the ability of male rats bearing MPOA lesions to mate. Indeed, about 50 per cent of the lesioned ergot-treated rats ejaculated, often after a low number of intromissions, and with short ejaculation latencies (Hansen *et al.* 1982*a*). Daily injections with naloxone, by contrast, were not effective (Hansen *et al.* 1982*a*).

There is at present uncertainty as to the neurochemical mechanism underlying lisuride's potent behavioural actions, its effect in other, but related models, having been blocked by depletion of endogeneous monoamines or by the administration of DA receptor blockers or 5-HT receptor agonists (Horowski and Darow 1981). Nor is much known about lisuride's site of action, although a recent study suggests that the selective exposure of the spinal cord to lisuride, by way of intrathecal injections, is as effective as systemic injections in facilitating the mating behaviour of neurologically intact rats (Hansen 1982). Further studies on the mechanism by which lisuride activates sexual behaviour in MPOA lesioned animals are clearly needed, and may reveal the existence of monoaminergic links between hormone-sensitive neurones in the hypothalamus and spinal genito-pelvic reflex systems involved in copulation.

References

Alton, E. F. W., Wright, Ch., and Everitt, B. J. (1979). Catecholamine mechanisms in the hormonal regulation of sexual behaviour. In *Catecholamines: basic and clinical frontiers* (eds. E. Usdin, I. Kopin, and J. Barchas) vol. II, pp. 1766–7. Plenum Press, New York.

Barfield, R. J., Wilson, C. A., and McDonald, P. G. (1975). Sexual behaviour: extreme reduction of postejaculatory refractory period by midbrain lesions in male rats. *Science* **189**, 147–9.

Baum, M. J. and Starr, M. S. (1980). Inhibition of sexual behaviour by dopamine antagonists or serotonin agonist drugs in castrated male rats given estradiol or dihydrotestosterone. *Pharmac. Biochem. Behav.* **13**, 57–67.

Caggiula, A. R., Shaw, D. H., Antelman, S. M., and Edwards, D. J. (1976). Interactive effects of brain catecholamines and variations in sexual and nonsexual arousal on copulatory behaviour of male rats. *Brain Res.* **111**, 321–36.

— — Antelman, S. R., Chiodo, L. A., and Lineberry, C. G. (1979*a*). Brain dopamine and sexual behaviour. Psychopharmacological and electrophysiological evidence for an antagonism between active and passive components. In *Catecholamines: Basic and clinical frontiers* (eds. E. Usdin, I. Kopin, and J. Barchas) vol. II, pp. 1766–7. Plenum Press, New York.

— — Hernden, J. G., Scanlon, R., Greenstone, D., Bradshaw, W., and Sharp, D. (1979*b*). Dissociation of active from immobility components of sexual behaviour in female rats by central 6-hydroxydopamine: implications for CA involvement in sexual behaviour and sensorimotor responsiveness. *Brain Res.* **172**, 505–20.

Chiodo, L. A., Caggiula, A. R., Antelman, S. H., and Lineberry, C. G. (1979). Reciprocal influences of activating and immobilizing stimuli on the activity of nigrostriatal dopamine neurons. *Brain Res.* **176**, 385–90.

Christensen, L. W. and Clemens, L. G. (1974). Intrahypothalamic implants of testosterone or estradiol and resumption of masculine sexual behaviour in long-term castrated male rats. *Endocrinology* **95**, 984–90.

Clark, T. K. (1980). Male rat sexual behaviour compared after 6-OHDA and electrolytic lesions in the dorsal NA bundle region of the midbrain. *Brain Res.* **202**, 429–43.

—— Caggiula, A. R., McConnell, R. A., and Antelman, S. M. (1975). Sexual inhibition is reduced by rostral midbrain lesions in the male rat. *Science NY* **190**, 169–71.

Davidson, J. M. (1966). Activation of the male rat's sexual behaviour by intra-cerebral implantation of androgen. *Endocrinology* **79**, 783–94.

Davis, P. G., McEwen, B. S., and Pfaff, D. W. (1979). Localized behavioural effects of tritiated estradiol implants in the ventromedial hypothalamus of female rats. *Endocrinology* **104**, 898–903.

Everitt, B. J. (1978). A neuroanatomical approach to the study of monoamines and sexual behaviour. In *Biological determinants of sexual behaviour* (ed. J. B. Hutchison) pp. 555–74. Wiley, Chichester.

—— Fuxe, K., and Hokfelt, T. (1974). Inhibitory role of dopamine and 5-hydroxytryptamine in the sexual behaviour of female rats. *Eur. J. Pharmac.* **29**, 187–91.

—— —— —— and Jonsson, G. (1976). Role of monoamines in the control by hormones of sexual receptivity in the female rat. *J. Comp. Physiol. Psychol.* **89**, 556–72.

Hansen, S. (1982). Spinal control of sexual behaviour: effects of intrathecal administration of lisuride. (Submitted).

—— and Ross, S. B. (1982). Role of descending monoaminergic neurons in the control of sexual behaviour: effects of intrathecal infusions of 6-hydroxy-dopamine and 5,7-dihydroxytryptamine. (Submitted).

—— and Sodersten, P. (1979). Reversal of progesterone inhibition of sexual behaviour in ovariectomized rats by high doses of progesterone. *J. Endocrinol.* **80**, 381–8.

—— Köhler, Ch., Goldstein, M., and Steinbusch, H. V. M. (1982*a*). Effects of ibotenic acid-induced neuronal degeneration in the medial preoptic area and the lateral hypothalamic area on sexual behaviour in the male rat. *Brain Res.* **239**, 213–32.

—— —— —— (1982*b*). On the role of the dorsal mesencephalic tegmentum in the control of masculine sexual behaviour in the rat: effects of electrolytic lesions, ibotenic acid and DSP4. *Brain Res.* **240**, 311–20.

—— Stanfield, E. J., and Everitt, B. J. (1980). The role of ventral bundle nor-adrenergic neurons in sensory components of sexual behaviour and coitus induced pseudopregnancy. *Nature, Lond.* **286**, 152–4.

—— —— —— (1981). The effects of lateral tegmental noradrenergic neurons on components of sexual behaviour and pseudopregnancy in female rats. *Neuroscience* **6**, 1105–17.

Hebb, D. O. (1955). Drives and the C.N.S. (Conceptual Nervous System). *Psychol. Rev.* **62**, 243–54.

Heritage, A. S., Grant, L. D., and Stumpf, W. E. (1977). ^{3}H-estradiol in catechol-amine neurons of the rat brain stem; combined localization by autoradiography and formaldehyde-induced fluorescence. *J. Comp. Neurol.* **176**, 607–30.

Hitt, J. C., Hendricks, S. E., Ginsberg, S. I., and Lewis, J. H. (1970). Disruption of male, but not female, sexual behaviour in rats by medial forebrain bundle lesions. *J. Comp. Physiol. Psychol.* **73**, 377–84.

Horowski, R. and Dorow, R. (1981). Influence of estradiol and other gonadal steroids on central effects of lisuride and comparable ergot derivatives. In *Gonadal steroids and brain function* (eds. W. Wuttke and R. Horowski), *Exp. 1 Brain Res.* Suppl. 3, pp. 169–81.

Jonsson, G. (1980). Chemical neurotoxins as denervation tools in neurobiology. *Ann Rev. Neurosci.* **3**, 169–87.

Keverne, E. B. and de la Riva, C. (1982). Pheromones in mice: reciprocal interaction between the nose and brain. *Nature, Lond.* **296**, 142–50.

—— Poindron, P., Levy, F., and Lindsay, D. R. (1982). Vaginal stimulation: an important determinant of maternal bonding in sheep. *Science NY* **219**, 81–3.

Lindvall, O. and Bjorklund, A. (1978). Organization of catecholamine neurons in the rat central nervous system. In *Handbook of psychopharmacology* (eds. L. L. Iversen, S. D. Iversen and S. H. Snyder), vol. 9, pp. 139–231. Plenum Press, New York.

Malmnäs, C. O. (1973). Monoaminergic influence on testosterone-activated copulatory behaviour in the castrated male rat. *Acta Physiol. Scand. Suppl.* 395.

Meyersen, B. J. and Malmnäs, C. O. (1978). Brain monoamines and sexual behaviour. In *Biological determinants of sexual behaviour* (ed. J. B. Hutchison) pp. 521–54. Wiley, Chichester.

McEwen, B. S., Davis, P. G., Parsons, B., and Pfaff, D. W. (1979). The brain as a target for steroid hormone action. *Ann. Rev. Neurosci.* **2**, 65–112.

Mogenson, G. J. and Phillips, A. G. (1976). Motivation: a psychological construct in search of a physiological substrate. In *Progress in psychobiology and physiological psychology* (eds. J. M. Sprague and A. N. Epstein) pp. 189–243. Academic Press, New York.

Moore, R. Y. (1980). The reticular formation: monoamine neuron systems. In *The reticular formation revisited* (eds. J. A. Hobson and M. A. B. Brazier) pp. 67–81. Raven Press, New York.

Nauta, W. J. H. and Haymaker, W. (1969). Hypothalamic nuclei and fiber connections. In *The hypothalamus* (eds. W. Haymaker, E. Anderson and W. J. H. Nauta) pp. 136–209. Thomas, Springfield.

Paglietti, E., Pellegrini-Quarantotti, B., Merev, G., and Gessa, G. L. (1978). Apomorphine and l-dopa lower ejaculation threshold in the male rat. *Physiol. Behav.* **20**, 559–62.

Parsons, C. E., Stanfield, E., Hansen, S., and Everitt, B. J. (1981). Effects of lateral tegmental noradrenergic neuron lesions, and infusion of noradrenaline in the ventral tegmental area on sexual and open field behaviour in female rats. *J. Anat.* **133**, 118.

Pfaff, D. W. and Sakuma, Y. (1979). Deficit in the lordosis reflex of female rats caused by lesions in the ventromedial nucleus of the hypothalamus. *J. Physiol.* **228**, 203–10.

Robbins, T. W. and Everitt, B. J. (1982). Functional studies of central catecholamines. *Int. Rev. Neurobiol.* **23**, 303–65.

Rubin, B. S. and Barfield, R. J. (1980). Priming of estrous responsiveness by implants of 17 β estradiol in the ventromedial hypothalamic nucleus of female rats. *Endocrinology* **106**, 504–9.

—— —— (1981). Site of action of progesterone in the regulation of estrous responsiveness in female rats. *Proc. of the Conference on Reproductive Behavior, Vanderbilt University, Nashville, Tennessee*, p. 25. Vanderbilt University, Nashville.

Schwarcz, R., Hökfelt, T., Fuxe, K., Jonsson, G., Goldstein, M., and Terenius, L. (1979). Ibotenic acid-induced neuronal degeneration: a morphological and neurochemical study. *Exp. Brain Res.* **37**, 199–216.

Slimp, J. C., Hart, B. L., and Goy, R. W. (1978). Heterosexual, autosexual and social behavior of adult rhesus monkeys with medial preoptic-anterior hypothalamic lesions. *Brain Res.* **142**, 105–22.

Stellar, E. (1954). The physiology of motivation. *Psychol. Rev.* **61**, 5–22.

Swanson, L. W. and Mogenson, G. J. (1981). Neural mechanisms for the functional coupling of autonomic endocrine and somatomotor responses in adaptive behavior. *Brain Res. Rev.* **3**, 1–34.

This research was supported by the British Medical Research Council (Grant No. PG733722, BJE), the Bank of Sweden Tercentenary Foundation, and the Swedish Medical Research Council (SH).

2

Dopamine receptors and premature ejaculation

GIAN LUIGI GESSA AND LUCIA NAPOLI-FARRIS

INTRODUCTION

ALTHOUGH premature ejaculation (ejaculatio praecox) is one of the most frequent human sexual dysfunctions, being as old as mankind and disturbing not only for the male sufferer but also for his partner, there are no studies, to our knowledge, on the neurochemical substrate involved in this condition; the interpretation of it being essentially psychological. The reasons for this silence might be attributed to the lack of suitable animal models. Yet, marked shortening of ejaculation threshold may normally occur or may be pharmacologically induced in the laboratory rat. In fact, among a population of sexually experienced male rats, some subjects may be found which ejaculate after much fewer penile intromissions and after much shorter latency, than the majority of animals of the same strain. Besides this 'natural' model of premature ejaculation, the latter may be produced in rats by the administration of different dopamine (DA) receptor stimulants.

INFLUENCES ON SEXUAL FUNCTIONS

This chapter is intended to provide evidence that (a) DA receptors responsible for pharmacologically induced premature ejaculation have similar characteristics to DA autoreceptors or may be identified with them, and (b) that such receptors may play an important role in regulating erection and ejaculation mechanisms. In this contribution, receptors are intended as a functional entity, leaving the problem of their molecular and anatomical characterization unresolved.

Definition of DA autoreceptors

There is good evidence to indicate that a special kind of DA receptor in the central nervous system (CNS) is located on the dopaminergic neurone itself, in the somatodendritic region or presynaptically on dopaminergic terminals (Bunney, Walters, Roth, and Aghajanian 1973; Carlsson 1975; Roth 1979). The stimulation of such receptors would result in decreased dopaminergic firing, and reduced DA synthesis and release. A characteristic of DA autoreceptors is considered to be that of being more sensitive to DA agonists, than postsynaptic DA receptors located on the effector cells responsible for stimulatory motor responses (Skirboll, Grace, and Bunney 1979). Therefore, doses of apomorphine and other DA receptor stimulants needed to stimulate DA autoreceptors, are much lower than those needed to produce stereotypy and motor stimulation. Recently, a rather selective stimulant for DA autoreceptors has been synthetized, 3-(3-hydroxyphenyl)-*N-n*-propylpiperidine (3-PPP) (Hjorth, Carlsson, Wikström, Lindberg, Sanchez, Hacksell, Arvidsson, Svensson, and Nilsson 1981). As reported below, this compound might prove to be an important chemical tool for elucidating the possible nature of the receptors involved in the sexual stimulant response to DA agonists.

Erection and ejaculation

Minute doses of direct or indirect DA receptor stimulants such as apomorphine, *N-n*-propyl-norapomorphine (NPA), amphetamine, amantadine, and lisuride produce repeated episodes of penile erection, sometimes followed by ejaculation in adult male rats. These may occur in isolation or in groups with other males (Baraldi and Bertolini 1974; Baraldi and Benassi-Benelli 1975; Benassi-Benelli, Ferrari, and Pellegrini-Quarantotti 1979). The sexual response to DA agonists is due to the stimulation of central DA receptors, since it is prevented by centrally acting DA receptor blockers, but not by domperidone, a DA blocker which does not cross the blood–brain barrier (Benassi-Benelli *et al.* 1979).

Doses of DA agonists required to elicit the sexual response are much lower than those necessary to elicit hyperactivity and stereotypy. NPA is by far the most potent compound to induce penile erection, the minimum active dose being in the order of a few micrograms per kilogram. Apomorphine and NPA produce a bell-shaped dose-response curve: in that their effect is proportional to the dose up to a maximum active dose. After that higher doses are progressively less effective until the stimulant response ceases, and finally even the normal occurrence of penile erection is suppressed.

The reason for the inhibitory effect of the high doses is not clear. Since the stimulant effect of apomorphine on penile erection ceases when the dose is high enough to elicit stereotypy, it was suggested that activation of DA receptors sustaining the latter response would oppose that of receptors producing penile erection. However, since NPA, unlike apomorphine, is maximally effective in eliciting penile erection in doses that also cause a high degree of stereotypy, this explanation is no longer tenable. On the other hand, it was found that naloxone, an opiate receptor antagonist, reverses the inhibitory effect of the higher doses of apomorphine and NPA on penile erection, suggesting that overstimulation of DA receptors results in the release of opiate peptides which tend to dampen sexual stimulant response (Ferrari and Baggio 1982).

MECHANISMS OF DA EFFECTS

Premature ejaculation and DA agonists

Selected sexually experienced rats attain ejaculation with receptive females after 8–13 penile intromissions into the vagina, and within 8–12 min after the first intromission. 'Premature ejaculation' in rats can be defined as a decrease in both the number of intromissions preceding ejaculation (intromission frequency) and the time interval between the first intromission and the first ejaculation (ejaculation latency): ejaculation refers to the behavioural response and not to seminal emission.

TABLE 2.1 *Decreased ejaculation threshold caused by dopamine receptor stimulants in rats*

Treatment (30 min before test)	mg/kg		EF	IF	EL
Saline	–		2.5 ± 0.3	13.1 ± 1.5	898.0 ± 141
Apomorphine	0.05	s.c.	2.3 ± 0.4	5.5 ± 1.1*	539.1 ± 92*
NPA	0.0025	s.c.	2.8 ± 1.3	4.6 ± 1.8*	680.3 ± 13*
L-DOPA	100	i.p.	1.8 ± 0.3	8.0 ± 0.8*	570.3 ± 110*
3-PPP	10	s.c.	2.1 ± 0.8	6.2 ± 1.3*	760.5 ± 180*
Lisuride	0.4	i.p.	3.9 ± 0.2*	6.2 ± 1.3*	520.6 ± 87*

Each value is the mean ± SE of at least six animals.
EF = ejaculation frequency; IF = intromission frequency; EL = ejaculation latency (s); 3-PPP = (+)3-(3-hydroxyphenyl-*N-n*-propylpiperidine).

Table 2.1 shows that the administration of apomorphine, NPA, L-DOPA, 3-PPP, and lisuride, given to the male rat 30 min prior to the mating test with the receptive female, markedly decrease the number of intromissions prior to ejaculation and shorten ejaculation latency (Paglietti, Pellegrini-Quarantotti, Mereu, and Gessa 1977; Gessa, Benassi-Benelli, Falaschi, and Ferrari 1980). Doses of DA agonists necessary to elicit premature ejaculation are the same as those that produce penile erection. Accordingly, NPA is the most potent DA agonist, the active dose being as low as 2.5/µg/kg subcutaneously. Moreover, doses of DA agonists producing premature ejaculation are within the dose range that is needed to activate DA autoreceptors, but much lower than those needed to produce stereotypy and motor stimulation.

These results suggest that DA receptors responsible for premature ejaculation and penile erection might be identified with the DA autoreceptors or have close similarities with the latter.

The effect of lisuride has been attributed by Ahlenius, Larsson, and Svensson (1980) to the impairment of brain serotonin (5-HT) neurotransmission, secondary to the stimulation of 5-HT autoreceptors. They have argued that similar decreases in intromission frequency and ejaculation latency are produced by *p*-chlorophenylalanine (PCPA) Salis and Dewsbury 1971), an inhibitor of 5-HT synthesis, and that lisuride is a more potent agonist for 5-HT receptors than for DA receptors. Although a possible involvement of 5-HT receptors in premature ejaculation cannot be excluded at present, several arguments favour the DA autoreceptor hypothesis. Doses of lisuride needed to modify sexual pattern are far higher than those required to suppress 5-HT firing by 5-HT autoreceptor stimulation (Rogawski and Aghajanian 1979), and PCPA does not selectively inhibit the synthesis of 5-HT but partially inhibits also that of catecholamines (Tagliamonte, Tagliamonte, Corsini, Mereu, and Gessa 1973). On the other hand, interference with 5-HT neurotransmission may explain the fact that lisuride, similarly to PCPA, increases the number of ejaculations during the observation period (Table 2.1) and reinduces full copulatory behaviour in castrated male rats (Ahlenius *et al.*, 1980).

Impairment of DA neurotransmission

3-PPP is one of the DA agonists found to reduce ejaculation threshold. This compound has been shown to be a rather selective stimulant of DA autoreceptors. In fact, unlike apomorphine and NPA, it fails, even at the highest doses, to evoke any response associated with postsynaptic DA receptor stimulation (Hjorth *et al.* 1981). These results suggest that premature ejaculation is produced by the activation of DA autoreceptors and the secondary inhibition of DA neurotransmission.

This hypothesis is supported by the results reported in Table 2.2, showing that haloperidol, but not domperidone, produces a marked decrease in intromission frequency. In fact, as expected from previous studies (Gessa and Taglia-

TABLE 2.2 *Effect of haloperidol on copulatory behaviour in the male rat*

Haloperidol (mg/kg i.p.)	h after treatment	% animals achieving ejaculation	EF	IF	EL
None	–	100	3.4 ± 0.3	10.8 ± 1.9	367 + 30
0.1	1	80	3.2 ± 0.2	9.1 ± 1.1	385 + 40
0.25	1	20*	–	–	–
0.25	3	100	3.1 ± 0.1	4.1 ± 0.5*	340 + 60
1.00	1	10*	–	–	–
1.00	6	85	3.0 ± 0.2	5.3 ± 0.2*	381 + 35

Each value is the mean ± SE of 12 rats.

monte 1974), 1 h after haloperidol treatment, copulatory behaviour was suppressed in about 80 per cent of the animals. However, unexpectedly, 6 h after treatment, in spite of the presence of marked catalepsy, almost all of the animals resumed copulation. However, in these rats ejaculation occurred after much fewer intromissions than normal. The haloperidol effect differs from that of DA agonists in that it does not reduce the ejaculation latency. However, one should consider that the neurological deficit produced by the neuroleptic might interfere with the animals' ability to perform the copulatory act. It is not clear why haloperidol suppresses copulatory behaviour during the first hour after treatment, with disappearance of the inhibition later when the neuroleptic effect is maximal. A detailed study on the effect of DA receptor blockade on various components of copulatory behaviour might shed some light on this problem.

Putative role of ACTH and MSH

We found that penile erection as well as the repeated yawning induced by apomorphine are prevented by cycloheximide, the time-course of the inhibition paralleling the inhibitory effect on brain protein synthesis (Serra, Fratta, Collu, Napoli-Farris, and Gessa 1982). This suggests that a newly synthetized peptide is needed for apomorphine response, and ACTH or MSH peptides might be possible candidates for mediating such an effect. In fact, the injection of microgram quantities of these peptides into the cerebrospinal fluid (CSF) of different mammals causes recurrent episodes of penile erection and ejaculation, associated with repeated yawning (Bertolini, Vergogni, Gessa, and Ferrari 1969). The latter is also produced by apomorphine and NPA.

In rabbits, which are most sensitive to the sexual effect of ACTH and MSH peptides, sexual stimulation may be so intense that, during the first 2 or 3 h following treatment, the animals may ejaculate up to a dozen times. As shown in Table 2.3, the administration of $ACTH_{1-24}$ or α-MSH into the lateral ventricle

TABLE 2.3 *Decreased ejaculation threshold in rats after $ACTH_{1-24}$ and α-MSH*

Treatment (30 min before test)	μg i.c.v.	EF	IF	EL
Saline	10	2.8 ± 0.4	9.0 ± 0.5	980.5 ± 111
$ACTH_{1-24}$	5	3.1 ± 0.3	5.3 ± 0.7*	525.6 ± 75*
α-MSH	2.5	3.3 ± 0.4	5.1 ± 0.3*	495.7 ± 130*

Each value is the mean ± SE of 12 animals, chronically implanted with a cannula in the lateral ventricle (Bertolini *et al.*, 1969).

of sexually experienced male rats, copulating with receptive females, markedly shortens the ejaculation latency and also decreases the number of intromissions prior to ejaculation (Bertolini, Gessa, and Ferrari 1975). The peptidic sequence necessary to induce erection and ejaculation is that of $ACTH_{1-12}$: present in natural ACTH, α- and β-MSH and β-LPH (see Bertolini and Gessa 1981). No other peptide, including LHRH is capable of producing a similar response.

On the basis of these results, we might suggest that stimulation of DA autoreceptors results in the release of MSH or ACTH peptides from pituitary, or from peptidergic neurones in the brain. It is pertinent to recall that MSH-producing cells in the intermediate lobe of the hypophysis are under the inhibitory control of dopaminergic neurones originating from the arcuate nucleus of the hypothalamus (Jackson, Hope, Estivariz, and Lowry 1981).

CONCLUSIONS

A model of premature ejaculation can be produced in rats by the administration of DA agonists. Premature ejaculation is defined as the stage at which the animal achieves ejaculation with a receptive female, after fewer intromissions and shorter latency than normal. Doses of DA agonists producing premature ejaculation are within the dose range needed for stimulating DA autoreceptors, i.e. those receptors whose stimulation results in the inhibition of DA neurotransmission.

These results indicate the existence in the CNS of a special kind of DA receptor which regulates ejaculation threshold. The nature of these receptors is not established. The findings presented suggest that they might be identified with DA autoreceptors and that premature ejaculation is the result of an impairment of DA neurotransmission in some brain region. Consistently, premature ejaculation is elicited by 3-PPP, a rather selective stimulant of DA autoreceptors.

Moreover, 6 h after haloperidol treatment, rats achieve ejaculation after fewer intromissions than normal.

Alternatively, it is possible that DA receptors involved in the sexual response to apomorphine and other DA agonists, might consist of a special kind of postsynaptic DA receptor, more sensitive to the agonists than those receptors responsible for stereotypy, motor stimulation, and EEG arousal. Finally, the apparent high sensitivity of DA receptors responsible for the sexual effect, might depend on the fact that they are more accessible to DA agonists across the blood–brain barrier.

Apart from their nature and anatomical location, the finding that a special population of DA receptors may be involved in premature ejaculation, might offer new ideas to control such disturbance occurring in man. According to our hypothesis, drugs which preferentially block such receptors should be useful in premature ejaculation. It is possible that the therapeutic efficacy on this condition observed with thioridazine (Singh 1963) and metoclopramide (Falaschi, Rocco, De Giorgio, Frajese, Fratta, and Gessa 1981) might be due to such a mechanism.

References

Ahlenius, S., Larsson, K., and Svensson, L. (1980). Stimulating effects of lisuride on masculine sexual behaviour of rats. *Eur. J. Pharmac.* **64**, 47–51.

Baraldi, M. and Bertolini, A. (1974). Penile erections induced by amantadine in male rats. *Life Sci.* **14**, 1231–35.

—— and Benassi-Benelli, A. (1975). Induzione di erezioni ripetute nel ratto adulto mediante apomorfina. *Riv. Farmacol. Terap.* **VI**, 147–9.

Benassi-Benelli, A., Ferrari, F., and Pellegrini-Quarantotti, B. (1979). Penile erection induced by apomorphine and *N-n*-propylnorapomorphine in rats. *Arch. Int. Pharmacodyn.* **241**, 128–34.

Bertolini, A., Vergogni, W., Gessa, G. L., and W. Ferrari (1969). Induction of sexual excitement by the action of adrenocorticotrophic hormone in brain. *Nature, Lond.* **221**, 667–9.

—— and Gessa, G. L. (1981). Behavioural effects of ACTH and MSH peptides. *J. Endocrinol. Invest.* **4**, 241–51.

—— —— and Ferrari, W. (1975). Penile erection and ejaculation: A central effect of ACTH-like peptides in mammals. In *Sexual behaviour: pharmacology and biochemistry* (eds. M. Sandler and G. L. Gessa) pp. 247–57. Raven Press, New York.

Bunney, B. S., Walters, J. R., Roth, R. H. and Aghajanian, G. K. (1973). Dopaminergic neurons: Effect of antipsychotic drugs and amphetamine on single cell activity. *J. Pharmacol. Exp. Ther.* **185**, 560–4.

Carlsson, A. (1975). Receptor-mediated control of dopamine metabolism. In *Pre and post synaptic receptors* (eds. E. Usdin and W. E. Bunney) pp. 49–63, Marcel Dekker, New York.

Falaschi, P., Rocco, A., De Giorgio, G., Frajese, G., Fratta, W., and Gessa, G. L. (1981). Brain dopamine and premature ejaculation: Results of treatment with dopamine antagonists. In *Apomorphine and other dopaminomimetics* (eds. G. L. Gessa and G. U. Corsini) Vol. 1, pp. 117–21. Raven Press, New York.

Ferrari, F. and Baggio, G. (1982) Potentiation of the aphrodisiac effect of *N-n*-propyl-norapomorphine by naloxone. *Eur. J. Pharmac.* **81**, 321–6.

Gessa, G. L., Benassi-Benelli, A., Falaschi, P., and F. Ferrari (1980). Role of dopamine in erection and ejaculation mechanisms. In *Endocrinology 1980* (eds. I. A. Cummings, G. W. Funder, and F. A. O. Mendelsohn) pp. 619–21. *Proc. Aust. Acad. Sci.*

— — and Tagliamonte, A. (1974). Possible role of brain serotonin and dopamine controlling male sexual behaviour. *Adv. Biochem. Psychopharmac.* **11**, 217–27.

Hjorth, S., Carlsson, A., Wikström, H., Lindberg, P., Sanchez, D., Hacksell, U., Arvidsson, L., Svensson, U., and Nilsson, J. L. G. (1982). 3-PPP, a new centrally acting DA-receptor agonist with selectivity for autoreceptors. *Trends Pharmac. Sci.* **3**, 232.

Jackson, S., Hope, J., Estivariz, F., and Lowry, P. J. (1981). Nature and control of peptide release from the pars intermedia. In *Peptides of the Pars Intermedia*, pp. 141–62. Pitman, London.

Paglietti, E., Pellegrini-Quarantotti, B., Mereu, G., and Gessa, G. L. (1978). Apomorphine and L-DOPA lower ejaculation threshold in the male rat. *Physiol. Behav.* **20**, 599–62.

Rogawski, M. A. and Aghajanian, G. K. (1979). Response of central monoaminergic neurons to lisuride: comparison with LSD. *Life Sci.* **24**, 1289–98.

Roth, R. H. (1979). Dopamine autoreceptors: Pharmacology function and comparison with postsynaptic dopamine receptors. *Commun. Psychopharmac.* **3**, 429–45.

Salis, P. G. and Dewsbury, D. A. (1971). Para-chlorophenylalanine facilitates copulatory behaviour in male rats. *Nature, Lond.* **323**, 400–2.

Serra, G., Fratta, W., Collu, M., Napoli-Farris, L., and Gessa, G. L. (1982). Cycloheximide prevents apomorphine induced yawning, penile erection and genital grooming in rats. *Eur. J. Pharmac.* (in press).

Singh, H. (1963). Therapeutic use of thioridazine in premature ejaculation. *Am. J. Psychiat.* **119**, 891.

Skirboll, L. R., Grace, A. A., and Bunney, B. S. (1979). Dopamine auto- and postsynaptic receptors: Electrophysiological evidence for differential sensitivity to dopamine agonists. *Science* **206**, 80–2.

Tagliamonte, A., Tagliamonte, P., Corsini, G. U., Mereu, G. P., and Gessa, G. L. (1973). Decreased conversion of tyrosine to catecholamines in the brain of rats treated with *p*-chlorophenylalanine. *J. Pharm. Pharmac.* **25**, 101–3.

3
Serotonin and sexual behaviour

J. C. TUCKER AND SANDRA E. FILE

INTRODUCTION

THERE ARE at least five ways in which serotonin (5-HT) could influence sexual behaviour. First, specific 5-HT pathways might modify sexual behaviour quite independently of any hormonal influence on that behaviour. Secondly, 5-HT pathways might modify the hormonal milieu of the animal and thus alter sexual behaviour indirectly. Thirdly, sex hormones themselves might affect transmission in 5-HT pathways and this could then affect behaviour. Fourthly, the sensitivity of a behaviour to modification by 5-HT might depend on the animal being in a particular hormonal state, and might not be observed under otherwise identical conditions when the animal is not in this state. And finally, it is always important to consider that changes in sexual performance may be the indirect result of an effect of 5-HT on other behaviours — for instance changes in anxiety — or even the consequence of a completely general stimulation or sedation of the animal. This review will concentrate on the pharmacological manipulation of 5-HT function in the rat and the resulting changes in sexual behaviour; wherever possible the interaction with sex hormones will also be considered.

THE PHARMACOLOGICAL APPROACH

The classical, and most obvious, approach is to use drugs that will alter the function of serotonergic neurones. Table 3.1 summarizes the main classes of these drugs, with some examples of each class. It will be noted that there are disadvantages to this technique. Most of the available drugs lack specificity for 5-HT, and therefore actions on other transmitters are hard to exclude when postulating neural mechanisms. Furthermore, when administered systemically these drugs will affect all 5-HT receptors and thus it is always possible that actions at one site will be complicated, obscured, or even masked altogether by actions at another. It must also be taken into account that some drugs regarded as, say, antagonists at 5-HT receptors because they have that effect after direct application to the brain may not cross the blood–brain barrier at all well when they are given peripherally. In addition, of course, any peripheral actions must always be considered before one attributes a drug effect on behaviour to a central action of the drug. However, the net effects of drugs administered systemically have considerable clinical relevance. An alternative approach is to concentrate on specific anatomical 5-HT pathways and to destroy these by injection of neurotoxin or to make highly localized applications of drugs on to defined anatomical sites. Table 3.2 gives a summary of the main 5-HT pathways in the CNS.

TABLE 3.1 *Serotonergic agents: their desired and undesired effects*

Class of drug and name	Known drawbacks.
(1) Toxic agents	
Neurotoxins:	
5,6-Dihydroxytryptamine	General tissue damage
5,7-Dihydroxytryptamine	Damages NA neurones also
Vesicle-damaging depletors:	
Reserpine	Affects all amines
Tetrabenazine	Affects all amines
Release-enhancing depletors/synthesis inhibitors:	
p-Chlorophenylalanine (PCPA)	Transient 5-HT, NA release; short-term NA depletion; amino-acid transport inhibitor
p-Chloroamphetamine (pCA)	Neurotoxic metabolite(s)
p-Chloromethamphetamine	Affects catecholamines also
α-Propyldopacetamide	COMT, TyrOHase, and PheOHase inhibitor
Fenfluramine	Sedative
(2) Receptor agonists (also reduce 5-HT turnover)	
Lysergic acid di-ethylamide (LSD)	Dopamine agonist; peripheral antagonist(?)
5-Methoxy dimethyltryptamine	Increases NA turnover
Quipazine	Peripheral 5-HT antagonist; catecholamine agonist
Lisuride	Dopamine agonist
(3) Receptor antagonists (may be agonistic at low doses)	
Methysergide	Inhibits NA uptake; poor penetration to CNS
Methiothepin	DA and NA antagonist; poor penetration
Metergoline	Poor 5-HT but good tryptamine antagonism; DA agonist
Cinanserin	? Ineffective systemically
(4) Miscellaneous others	
Metabolic precursor:	
5-Hydroxytryptophan (5-HTP)	Can displace catecholamines
Re-uptake inhibitors:	
Clomipramine	Also affects NA uptake; histamine and acetylcholine antagonist
Zimelidine	Also affects NA *in vivo*
Monoamine oxidase inhibitors:	
Pargyline	Affects all amines
Nialamid	Affects all amines

TABLE 3.2a *A simplified description of the major serotonergic pathways in the CNS of the rat*

Gross area	Designation by Dahlstrom and Fuxe (1964)	Location of cell bodies*	Innervated targets
Medulla	B 1 B 2 B 3 B 4	R. pallidus R. obscurus R. magnus (ventral to IVth ventricle)	Ventral and dorsal horns of spinal cord ???
Pons	B 5 B 6	R. pontis (overlaps B 4)	Dorsal thalamus
Mid brain	B 7	R. dorsalis	Basal ganglia, s. nigra; amygdaloid nuclei, septo-hippocampal system, pyriform cortex, hypothalamus (see Part b)
	B 8	R. medianus	Cingulate cortex, septum, thalamus, olfactory tubercle, hypothalamus (see Part b)
	B 9	R. centralis sup.	caudate-putamen

*R. = raphe.
Sources: Dahlstrom and Fuxe (1964); Azmitia and Segal (1978).

TABLE 3.2b *The serotonergic innervation of hypothalamic areas*

Source (cell bodies)	Targets (if known)
Median raphe	Pre-optic area and anterior hypothalamus, arcuate nucleus, periventricular areas, lateral hypothalamus
Dorsal raphe	Arcuate nucleus, anterolateral areas
Paraventricular hypothalamus	Arcuate nucleus, ventromedial nucleus, dorsomedial areas, median eminence

Sources: Chan-Palay (1977); van de Kar and Lorens (1979).

Measurement of sexual behaviour

The experimental protocol that we use for work on the sexual behaviour of the male is based on those employed by Wilson and by Delini-Stula (personal communications). When combined with appropriate rearing conditions it will produce levels of sexual performance that are approximately in the middle range. This enables one to observe either enhancement or impairment of behaviour resulting from a particular drug treatment, without having to hypothesize in advance which may be the more likely result. Briefly, ovariectomized females are implanted with oestrogen and each male is exposed to a pair of these females.

Implants of oestradiol (oestra-1,3,5(10)triene-3,17-diol benzoic acid, melting point ca. 195°C) are made by dipping an entomological pin repeatedly into a pool of molten steroid. The exact size of the pellet is not crucial, since the technique relies for its effect on the slow but sustained release of oestrogen from a large depot: but the pins typically carry 25–30 mg of solid. The use of implants makes it unnecessary to inject the females repeatedly with oestrogen, and the level of circulating oestradiol that results is sufficient to induce receptivity in the overwhelming majority of females.

Preparation of the female

Adult females (ca. 200 g) are ovariectomized under barbiturate anaesthesia. At the time of surgery, a small incision is made in the scruff of the neck and the implant is inserted subcutaneously. After 7–10 days to recover from the surgery, the females should show signs of proceptivity, that is, soliciting behaviour (darting, hopping, ear-wiggling) when in the presence of a male. On being mounted, the lordosis posture is assumed, with the back flexed into a concave curve, the tail held to one side, and the neck extended. Alternatively, this behaviour can be produced by gently stroking the flanks of the female.

As a test arena we normally use an open-field apparatus 80 cm in diameter and 30 cm deep; it is helpful if the animals have enough room to chase each other, since this is an important part of the initiation phase of reproductive activity. The arena is indirectly illuminated by a 25 W deep red photographic safelight, to which rats are blind, and is situated in a quiet room away from other animals. Since the urine trails left by one rat may have marked effects on the behaviour of his successor (Stevens and Koster 1972; McIntosh, Davis, and Barfield 1979), we clean the arena after each trial using a little ethanol added to water.

Introduction of the male

The male to be tested is placed in the arena and allowed to explore it by himself for 5 min. After that time, a pair of receptive females are put in with him and the clock is re-started for the test proper. Normally, the immediate response on the male's part is an investigatory sniff, which should become prolonged when the female is in oestrus. In response, she will stretch her hind legs so that the anogenital region is held high off the floor. The observer then records the behaviour in the following categories. First, the times taken to initiate mounting (mount latency) and intromission: these two behaviours being distinguished by the fact that the dismount is almost a backward jump in the latter case. (The shorter of these two latencies is often referred to simply as the 'sexual latency'.) Then, individual mounts and intromissions are recorded until the male ejaculates, this being identified by an unusually long and deep intromission followed by a much slower dismount. The time is again noted at this point. The number of mounts and of intromissions required to reach ejaculation can then be counted.

The male then enters a refractory period in which he does not chase the females, and indeed often hardly moves at all; during this period he also produces an ultrasonic song, centred on around 22 kHz (Barfield and Geyer 1975), which can be made audible by means of a bat detector. The period during which the song is produced is termed the absolute refractory period, and the females tend to avoid him during this time. Eventually, the male revives and a new copulatory series is begun; it is interesting to consider that the females in fact control the temporal patterning of sexual interactions (McClintock 1974; Krieger, Orr, and Perper 1976). We usually terminate our trials 30 min after the introduction of the two females, during which time the more vigorous copulators will achieve three ejaculations, although two is a commoner figure.

There are two particular advantages to this methodology: first, latencies to mount can exceed 20 min when testing sluggish males, and secondly it also ensures that all males have had the same exposure to the females, even if the quality of the experience differs.

EXPERIMENTAL RESULTS

In this section we present some data that show how interaction with females when the male is juvenile can dramatically affect later sexual performance. Two specific types of interaction are likely to be important, namely interaction with the dam and interaction with female siblings. The results to be described originate from three groups of animals born in our laboratory. In every case, the pups were weaned on postnatal day 21 by removal of the dam. The males in Group 1 were reared in single-sex groups from birth, and consequently their dam was the only female they experienced. When they were tested for sexual behaviour, commencing in the twelfth postnatal week, they performed extremely poorly; in fact, not a single male mounted. In an attempt to stimulate at least some response, 15 males were selected and a single receptive female was left in the cage of each male overnight; the male was then re-tested, with a different female, on the following morning. However, even after two such overnight visits from different females, only four out of the 15 animals mounted in the ensuing test, and none of these reached an ejaculation or indeed displayed robust behaviour.

'Co-education' and the 'older woman' effect

The males in Group 2 had considerably more experience of females. Although they were kept in single-sex groups up to weaning, female pups of the same age were housed with the males from then on, in the proportion of roughly one female to every two males in the cage. We have termed this procedure 'co-educational rearing'. The females are removed in the eighth postnatal week, before their first oestrus about a week later. The important point is that they should be present for the adolescent play phase, since experiences during this period seem to lay the foundations of the adult patterns of behaviour and can indeed compensate for deficits acquired earlier in life (e.g. Shillito and Vogt 1978; Leedy, Vela, Popolow, and Gerall 1980).

In addition to co-education, these males were also exposed to mature oestrous females when they were still too young to show full adult behaviour, i.e. between days 35 and 40. At this stage the males weighed approximately 100 g while the females weighed approximately 180 g, and although no sexual behaviour as such was observed during this 5 min exposure, the results speak for themselves. The males were tested with the full protocol at between 10 and 13 weeks of age. In their first test, 40 out of 48 animals mounted successfully and three ejaculated, while in the second test a few days later 43 out of 47 mounted and 27 ejaculated.

The rats in Group 3 enabled us to discover whether co-education, or adolescent exposure, or both were responsible for the vast difference between Groups 1 and 2. The males of Group 3 were raised in the same style as those in Group 2, but did not receive exposure to an oestrous female before their first full test of sex. Twelve animals out of 32 mounted and six ejaculated, indicating that co-education alone has some effect but that the combination of treatments is considerably more potent. We have termed the increment in performance that results from adolescent exposure to mature oestrous females the 'older woman effect'.

The influence of the dam on later performance may be gauged from the

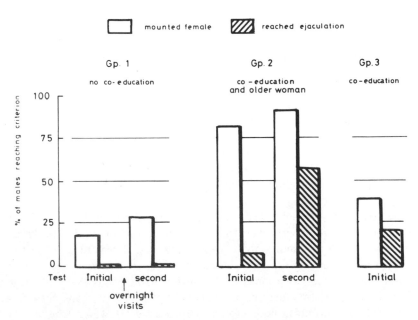

FIG. 3.1   The effects of juvenile heterosexual experience on sexual behaviours in adult rats. Group 1 rats received neither co-education nor experience of a mature, receptive female before testing. Between the first and second tests they entertained two receptive females in their home-cages on separate nights. Group 2 rats received both co-education (presence of female litter-mates in group-cage from weaning) and exposure to a mature, receptive female while adolescent. Group 3 rats received co-education but no experience of a mature, receptive female before testing.

results in a group of animals allocated at random to nine foster-mothers shortly after birth. By this means genetic effects should be completely controlled for, and any differences in performance between litters must result solely from postnatal experience. The postnatal experience of these pups was their dam, their co-educational partners, and their adolescent experience. We noted with some surprise that some litters nonetheless performed dramatically better in adult testing than others, and two of the most successful are compared with two of the most sluggish in Table 3.3.

TABLE 3.3   *The effects of foster-litter on sexual performance in adulthood. Comparison of two vigorous litters against two sluggish ones, from a total of nine*

	Vigorous litters		Sluggish litters	
	'A'	'I'	'B'	'C'
Latency to mount (s)	57	46	1118	542
Number of mounts in 30 min	23	33	10	25
Latency to first ejaculation (s)	519	862	1422	>1800

Environmental associations

There is good evidence that rats form long-term memories about their initial copulatory experiences (Thor and Holloway 1981), and we also have some interesting preliminary data on the way that performance in a test of sexual behaviour can be related to behaviour in other tests.

There were two independent groups of males in this study, each of which received a trial in a holeboard apparatus a few days after their sex test. However, one group had been tested for sexual behaviour actually in the holeboard box, albeit with a solid floor to cover the holes, while the second group had been tested in the open-field described above and the holeboard used was in a completely separate room.

The results of the holeboard experiments are shown in Table 3.4, having been divided into good performers (males that at least mounted the test females) and poor ones (those that did not). The sexually sluggish males had lower motor activity scores than the sexually successful males, regardless of the similarity between the two test environments ($F(1,56) = 4.48$, $P < 0.05$). This suggests that low motor activity may be a characteristic of, and perhaps even a contributing factor towards, poor sexual performance. However, the measures of exploration (number of dips and time spent head-dipping; File and Wardill 1975) were lower for the sexually sluggish males only when they were tested in the same apparatus for both experiments.

While no firm conclusions can be drawn from these preliminary data, we think that they raise the interesting possibilities that: (a) sexually sluggish males may be distinguished from vigorous males by more than just their sexual performance; and (b) the quality of sexual experience in a specific environment,

TABLE 3.4 *Behaviour of male rats in a holeboard apparatus 2 days after a test of sexual behaviour**

| | Sex experiment and holeboard experiment in | | | | | |
| | Same apparatus | | | Different apparatus | | |
Sexual performance	Number of head-dips	Duration	Motor activity	Number of head-dips	Duration	Motor activity
Success	22.0 ±1.9	21.7 ±2.1	270 ±28	20.8 ±2.4	20.0 ±1.9	302 ±11
		(n = 19)			(n = 12)	
No success	18.0 ±2.3	17.3 ±2.5	209 ±33	21.3 ±2.0	20.5 ±2.2	259 ±16
		(n = 11)			(n = 19)	

*Data shown separately for sexually successful and unsuccessful animals. One group received both tests in the same apparatus, while two different boxes were used for the other group.

For significance levels see text.

can affect other behaviours in that environment, presumably through a learned association with the apparatus cues.

SEXUAL NEURO-ANATOMY

Understanding of the anatomy of the serotonergic influence on sexual behaviour is emerging slowly. One location of considerable interest is the medial pre-optic area, which shades into the anterior hypothalamus without a clear boundary (Powers and Valenstein 1972). This region shows sexual dimorphism in its fine structure (Raisman and Field 1973), and appears to be one of the main projection areas for serotonergic fibres ascending from the midbrain (Grant and Stumpf, 1976; Azmitia 1978; van de Kar and Lorens 1979). It can be shown that stimulation of this area by implanted electrodes can enhance sexual function in the male (Malsbury 1971), even in castrates (van Dis and Larsson 1971). Destruction of the same region will inhibit the display of sexual behaviour (Heimer and Larsson 1966).

Yamanouchi (1980) reports the effects of lesions in the pre-optic area of female rats and his results support the view that descending fibres from an as yet uncertain, but non-hypothalamic source exert an inhibitory effect on the display of lordosis. This system is counteracted by a lordosis-facilitating system which can be damaged by cuts anterior to the ventromedial nucleus, by destruction of the ventromedial nucleus itself (Pfaff and Sakuma 1979b) or by isolation of the medio-basal hypothalamus (Yamanouchi 1980). Lesions of the pre-optic area can enhance lordosis (Nance, Christensen, Shryne, and Gorski 1977). Conversely, oestradiol implanted into the ventromedial nucleus will also cause animals to display enhanced lordosis (Barfield and Chen 1977; Mathews and Edwards 1977) and so will electrical stimulation (Pfaff and Sakuma 1979a). The existence of these two separate subsystems is mentioned at this point since it may help in the resolution of some of the conflicting data to be presented below. In addition, there has been a report of the discovery of cell bodies of serotonergic neurones located in the ventromedial hypothalamus (Chan-Palay 1977). Although the targets, and indeed the physiological function, of these cells have not yet been described the implications in relation to the effects of serotonin-altering drugs could be very important.

Unfortunately, a thorough discussion of the relevant neuro-anatomy lies outside the scope of this chapter, and the interested reader is therefore referred to the two or three papers cited here as convenient starting points.

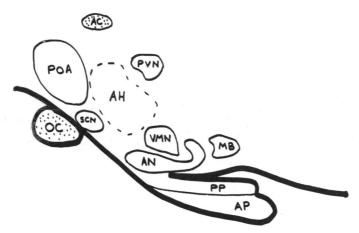

FIG. 3.2   A simplified para-sagittal view of the rat hypothalamus, indicating some locations relevant to sexual behaviour. Dotted areas indicate decussating fibre bundles: AC, anterior commissure; OC, optic chiasm. Gross anatomical regions: AH, anterior hypothalamic area; AP, anterior pituitary; MB, mammillary bodies; PP, posterior pituitary. Nuclei: AN, arcuate nucleus; POA, pre-optic area; PVN, para-ventricular nucleus; SCN, supra-chiasmatic nucleus; VMN, ventro-medial nucleus.

5HT AND THE MALE

Serotonin depletion and behaviour

There is a wealth of literature concerning the sexually stimulatory effects of the substance *p*-chlorophenylalanine (PCPA), which will severely deplete whole brain serotonin when given in fairly large doses. The depletion results from inhibition of the enzyme tryptophan hydroxylase, which performs the rate-determining step in the synthesis of serotonin from tryptophan. Independent work from three groups established that PCPA could facilitate mounting behaviour, both of females (Sheard 1969) and of other males (Shillito 1969), whilst Tagliamonte and several colleagues showed that PCPA facilitates both heterosexual and homosexual mounting under appropriate conditions. This effect of PCPA was enhanced by pargyline, a monoamine oxidase inhibitor, and could be prevented by injection of 5-hydroxytryptophan (5-HTP), the immediate precursor of 5-HT itself.

Behavioural effects are paralleled by reductions in brain 5-HT content (Tagliamonte, Tagliamonte, Gessa, and Brodie 1969; Gessa, Tagliamonte, Tagliamonte, and Brodie 1970, Tagliamonte, Tagliamonte, Stern, and Gessa 1970; Gessa, Tagliamonte, and Tagliamonte 1971). Several other workers have confirmed and expanded upon these results (e.g. Malmnäs and Meyerson, 1971; Salis and Dewsbury 1971). A note of dissent was sounded by Whalen and Luttge (1970), who failed to find any stimulation after PCPA, but their males were described as 'vigorous copulators' and it therefore seems likely that a ceiling effect was responsible (Gessa *et al.* 1971). Morden, Mullins, Levine, Cohen, and Dement (1968) divided rats into groups of low, middle, and high performers on the basis of screening tests and then applied chronic treatment with PCPA. Only the low-performance group responded to the drug. Similarly, Sjoerdsma, Lovenberg, Engelman, Carpenter, Wyatt, and Gessa (1970) tested what they termed 'sexually sluggish' males after treatment with PCPA or the monoamine oxidase inhibitor pargyline or the combination of the two. The last named treatment enabled all of the previously non-copulating males to perform successfully with receptive females. It is also possible to elicit lordotic responses from male rats primed with oestrogen, by using 5-HT depleting agents (Meyerson 1968; Larsson and Södersten 1971; Södersten and Ahlenius 1972) or 5-HT receptor blockers (Crowley, Ward, and Margules 1975).

   It should always be borne in mind that the effects of PCPA are not on 5-HT alone, and that it is therefore important to test the animals at a time when noradrenaline and dopamine would be expected to have recovered while 5-HT would still be depleted; this is typically 48–72 h after a single large dose. Sjoerdsma *et al.* investigated two of the known catabolites of PCPA, namely *p*-chlorophenylethylamine and *p*-chlorophenylpyruvate, but could find no evidence of stimulatory effects in male rats.

Return to baseline

Interestingly, the males used by Morden *et al.* (1968) apparently returned to their pre-drug baseline performance after withdrawal of PCPA, which in some ways is a rather surprising result; one might expect that some learning would have taken place. We recently carried out an experiment using 20 intact males treated with a single dose of 300 mg/kg PCPA or water, and tested 3 days later and again 1 week after that. In complete agreement with the published data on PCPA, we observed a marked enhancement of performance at the 3-day stage, when noradrenaline levels have recovered but 5-HT is still maximally depleted. As an example, the median mount latency of the PCPA males was 198 s as against 1208 s for the control ($P < 0.025$ by Mann–Whitney), and, in fact, several of the PCPA treated males achieved a third ejaculation in a 30-min test. However, an interesting feature of our data, which are shown in Fig. 3.3, is that the PCPA-treated males were still able to perform at a higher level than the controls after the 5-HT concentrations in their brains had fully recovered. For instance they still mounted much faster: the median latency was 188 s for the animals that had received PCPA and 1597 s for the controls

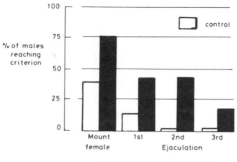
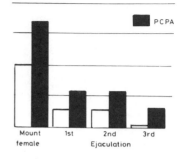

FIG. 3.3   The lasting effects of a single dose of PCPA (300 mg/kg) on sexual performance in previously sluggish male rats. The columns show the proportion of rats in each group (either PCPA or control) that achieved each of the criteria shown on the horizontal axis. The left-hand side shows the enhancement 3 days after injection, when 5-HT is maximally depleted; the right-hand side shows the enhancement 10 days after injection, when 5-HT levels are fully restored.

($P < 0.01$ by Mann–Whitney). It therefore seems likely that a rewarding sexual experience has lasting effects on performance, even when that experience was chemically induced.

The data we have presented extend the work by Ginton (1976), who also used non-copulating males. He found that animals that started to copulate 1 day after a 4-day course of PCPA (100 mg kg^{-1} day^{-1}) would continue to copulate even 8 weeks later. However, he subsequently treated all his control rats with PCPA also, and so it could not be determined whether the animals that originally received PCPA were still performing at higher levels than controls even after the serotonergic effects of the drug had worn off. We also confirm two of his incidental observations, namely that some rats completely fail to show stimulation after PCPA and that males that start to copulate after control injections will continue to do so in later tests. It would be of some interest to discover whether the performance of the formerly PCPA-treated males gradually decays back to control levels or whether they in fact remain more vigorous than controls indefinitely; a longer-term study than that reported here would be needed to determine this.

Toxin lesions

Serotonin neurones can be destroyed by the administration of the toxic di-hydroxy analogues of serotonin, although these also tend to affect cate-cholaminergic nerves to some extent. The rather unspecific neurotoxin, 5,6-dihydroxytryptamine (5,6-DHT), when given i.c.v., induced homosexual mounting behaviour in intact rats in the absence of females. (Da Prada, Carruba, O'Brien, Saner, and Pletscher 1972, *op. cit.*). Everitt (1977) and Larsson, Fuxe, Everitt, Holmgren, and Södersten (1978) used intracerebral 5,7-DHT, which is a more specific toxin for serotonergic cells, and did not observe this effect, although the lower dosages employed may have been responsible (Södersten,

Berge, and Hole 1978). Subsequently DaPrada *et al.* (1978) have reported finding an increase in both male–male mounting and in mounting by females after 5,6- or 5,7-DHT.

The role of testosterone

Gessa *et al.* (1970) reported that the presence of testosterone was required for PCPA to induce mounting, and although this was questioned by Mitler, Morden, Levine, and Dement (1972) and by Bond and co-workers (Bond, Shillito, and Vogt 1972) it later received support from other workers (del Fiaco, Fratta, Gessa, and Tagliamonte 1974). It is worth pointing out that all of the other studies mentioned so far were performed on intact males; it follows that the effects were observed in the presence of circulating testosterone, although changes in this hormone were not assessed. To avoid this difficulty, Malmnäs (1973) employed castrate males treated with a dose of testosterone that produced sub-maximal sexual performance, in order to confirm the role of 5-HT.

More recently, Södersten *et al.* (1978) carried out experiments to discover whether two treatments known to affect serotonin could be substituted for testosterone-replacement in the castrate male. Both 5,7-dihydroxytryptamine lesions and the depleting/lesioning agent *p*-chloroamphetamine (pCA) could restore the full repertoire of masculine sexual behaviours, from mounting to ejaculation, in their castrated rats; however, some males completely failed to respond to the treatments. When the same rats were tested again after being implanted with testosterone, the treated males still out-performed the animals whose serotonin levels had not been manipulated. Pre-treatment with zimelidine, which would prevent the pCA from entering the cell terminals, could also counteract pCA's behavioural effects. The depletions of 5-HT were assessed biochemically by measuring the loss of high-affinity re-uptake (Södersten *et al.* 1978). These results strengthen further their report (Södersten, Larsson, Ahlenius, and Engel 1976*a*) that PCPA could also restore full sexual vigour to castrated males, but only in 60 per cent of cases. The bimodal distribution of responses which they found seems to us to clarify the differences between the earlier papers discussed above.

Overall, then, it appears that depletion of serotonin has an invigorating effect on males that are sexually sluggish, but rather less or even no effect on males whose initial baseline activity is higher.

Serotonin agonists and antagonists

Reports on work using putative 5-HT receptor agonists provide almost the only indications of any complications in the relationship between 5-HT and masculine sexual behaviour. Following the hypothesis developed thus far, one would predict that these drugs would tend to inhibit sexual behaviour; in fact, they do the opposite. For instance, the ergot derivative lisuride stimulates mounting and shortens the ejaculatory latency (Da Prada, Bonetti, and Keller 1977; Ahlenius, Larsson, and Svensson 1980*a*), and certain experimental drugs derived from tetralins have similar effects. These consist of a reduction in the number of mounts and intromissions required before ejaculation is reached in intact males, and the facilitation even of sexual behaviour in castrated naive males, without maintaining doses of testosterone. However, the failure of the agonists LSD, quipazine, and 2,5-dimethoxy-4-methylamphetamine to affect sexual behaviour unless high doses were employed, has also been recorded (Ahlenius, Larsson, Svensson, Hjorth, Carlsson, Lindberg, Wikström, Sanchez, Arvidsson, Hacksell, and Nilsson 1981).

There seem to be only two straightforward explanations of these findings. One is that the compounds preferentially stimulate pre-synaptic, release-inhibiting autoreceptors (Aghajanian, Haigler and Bennett 1975; Rogawski and Aghajanian 1978). Alternatively they are, for some reason, acting as antagonists of 5-HT at the particular sites serving sexual behaviour. The third option, i.e. that the results observed do in fact result from postsynaptic 5-HT receptor stimulation, would entail disagreement with a large body of internally consistent work in many laboratories (including Ahlenius' own). There is the additional factor of the dopaminergic agonist activity of lisuride to consider. As for the tetralins, perhaps it can be remarked that here is an illustration of the difficulties one can encounter when using experimental substances which are claimed to be highly specific, but whose spectrum of action has not yet been understood in detail.

Re-uptake blockers

The drugs known as re-uptake inhibitors have the effect of blocking the high-affinity pumps located on synaptic membranes. These pumps serve to clear released transmitter from the cleft, and it follows that a block at this site leads, at least acutely, to an increase in the amount of neurotransmitter available to stimulate the postsynaptic receptors. One report in the literature has indicated that neonatal treatment with the tricyclic anti-depressant clomipramine, which is a serotonin re-uptake inhibitor, could adversely affect the sexual performance of the adult animals, even though the drug treatment ceased at weaning (Mirmiran, van de Poll, Corner, van Oyen, and Bour 1981). Thus the experimental animals were said both to intromit and ejaculate less often during a series of tests than did the controls, with a higher ratio of mounts to intromissions for each bout, although the latency to mount did not differ from the control values.

However, attempts to replicate these findings in our own laboratory have been wholly unsuccessful, (File and Tucker 1983), and in particular we have not found any combination of rearing and drug treatment conditions that would selectively impair sexual performance in the animals treated with clomipramine as pups (Table 3.5). We conclude that the results of Mirmiran *et al.* are an artefact, produced by their failure to use the split-litter, cross-fostered design that is appropriate for this type of study; the vital importance of this methodology is brought out strongly by the data presented in Table 3.3. Mirmiran's procedure fails to control for either genetic or rearing effects, and differences of the magnitude that we observed could easily create artefactual 'drug' effects when the control and the drug-treated animals belong to separate litters (Mirmiran *et al.*, op. cit.).

A number of re-uptake blockers available are considerably more selective

TABLE 3.5a *Sexual behaviour in adulthood after neonatal clomipramine*

Group	Control	Clomipramine		
	(n = 7)	3 mg/kg (n = 9)	10 mg/kg (n = 9)	30 mg/kg (n = 8)
Latency to to M or I	402 (17, >1800)	124 (39, >1800)	472 (16, 1742)	134 (57, 777)
Mounts	2.0 (0, 7)	3.2 (0, 28)	7.5* (0, 13)	6.5* (2, 17)
Intromissions	14.0 (0, 22)	15.0 (0, 24)	16.3 (1, 35)	14.0 (2, 28)
Latency to ejac. 1	1315 (347, >1800)	658 (460, >1800)	737 (538, > 1800)	690 (501, >1800)
Refractory period 1	510 (287, 510)	240 (97, 377)	315 (289, 359)	290 (270, 322)
Second copulatory series				
Mounts	0.5 (0, 1)	1.5 (0, 16)	3.6 (0, 5)	3.0 (0, 6)
Intromissions	8.5 (0, 10)	8.5 (0, 13)	9.5 (0, 13)	7.0 (0, 12)
Latency to ejac. 2	267 (195, 338)	252 (105, 804)	254 (158, 324)	284 (180, 406)
Refractory period 2	382 (350, 413)	406 (310, 504)	396 (285, 405)	389 (340, 448)

Median scores in each group, arranged by dose (values in parentheses show the range). All measures of time are quoted in seconds; test period was 1800 s.
Key: M, mount; I, intromission.
*Values show trend, but $P > 0.05$, Mann–Whitney test.

TABLE 3.5b *Proportion of males reaching several criteria*

Group	Control	Clomipramine		
		3 mg/kg	10 mg/kg	30 mg/kg
Proportion that mounted	6/7	8/9	9/9	8/8
Proportion that reached first ejaculation	4/7	6/9	6/9	4/8
Proportion that reached second ejaculation	2/5	6/9	4/7	4/8

for 5-HT pumps than is clomipramine. Hamburger-Bar, Rigter, and Dekker (1978) report the effects of the 5-HT-selective drug ORG 6582 on male sexual behaviour, as well as comparing it with both femoxetine and clomipramine. ORG 6582 and femoxetine both produced increases in sexual latency without changing the locomotor activity of the castrated, testosterone-maintained males that were employed; clomipramine had similar effects but these were significant only at one dose. The effects of ORG 6582 were still present 24 h after administration of the drug.

Ahlenius and his co-workers (Ahlenius *et al.* 1980*b*) used zimelidine and alaproclate to inhibit re-uptake. The drugs were administered in combination with benserazide: this substance inhibits the enzyme aromatic amino-acid decarboxylase and thus helps to ensure that the effects observed are indeed due to central 5-HT. They first pre-treated their males with a dose of 5-HTP that was insufficient to induce effects on sexual behaviour (12.5 mg/kg) in the absence of the re-uptake blocker. In the presence of the blocker, however, they observed prolonged ejaculation latencies and refractory periods. The 5-HTP + zimelidine combination also increased the frequency of intromission. When the blockers were tested in the absence of 5-HTP, zimelidine had no effects, although alaproclate alone was capable of increasing the number of mounts and prolonging the refractory period, in the same manner as had previously been shown for clomipramine (Ahlenius, Heimann, and Larsson 1979).

Steroid hormones

Baum and Starr (1980) studied the interaction of serotonin with the steroid hormones, a rather neglected area but probably one of great importance. The metobolic fate of testosterone involves conversion into oestradiol and 5α-dihydrotestosterone; one of the enzymes in the pathway has an aromatase activity. Using castrated males kept sexually active by testosterone, Christensen and Clemens (1975) had shown that the intracerebral administration of the aromatase blocker androst-1,4,6-triene-3,17-dione would also inhibit masculine sexual behaviour, in spite of the systemic presence of testosterone. It appears that oestradiol and 5α-dihydrotestosterone are essential for the expression of these behaviours, rather than the parent steroid. Further, Södersten *et al.* (1976*b*) had demonstrated that chronic treatment of castrated males with PCPA could maintain the entire repertoire of male sexual behaviour.

Baum and Starr built upon these findings. Castrated males were implanted peripherally with either oestradiol, dihydrotestosterone, or the combination of both; they then received the re-uptake inhibitor fluoxetine. The rates of mounting and intromission were reduced, with the most marked response in those animals loaded with both the steroids. Subsequently the same males were tested with the receptor agonist 5-methoxy-*N*,*N*-dimethyltryptamine. Unfortunately the small number of animals used for this experiment prevented the results from reaching significance, but their conclusions from the two experiments just discussed were that there was no detectable difference between oestradiol alone and dihydrotestosterone alone, but that animals treated with the combination were always more sensitive to serotonergic effectors than those treated with either steroid alone. They therefore proposed that one action of these two steroids was to suppress activity at serotonergic synapses.

Receptor antagonists

As part of the same series of experiments as those discussed above, Baum and Starr also investigated whether the receptor antagonist metergoline was able to counteract the effects of a much larger dose of 5-HTP (50 mg/kg), sufficient to produce clear-cut behavioural responses. In combination with benserazide this dose led to an increased number of mounts and intromissions before ejaculation, together with a prolongation of the ejaculatory latency and the refractory period. Although it had no effects when administered in the absence of ben-serazide + 5-HTP, a dose of 1 mg/kg of metergoline proved sufficient to abolish the effects resulting from the 5-HTP. These results are in accord with data from Benkert and Eversmann (1972) who showed that methysergide, another receptor antagonist of 5-HT, would stimulate sexual behaviour.

Shillito and Vogt (1978) observed no increase in mounting after treating both juvenile and adult males with methiothepin; however, this can most likely be attributed to the fact that methiothepin penetrates the blood–brain barrier only poorly.

5-HT AND THE FEMALE

On turning to the female, one finds that there is some doubt as to whether serotonin is involved at all in the control of the major sign of receptivity, i.e. lordosis. We start by considering the evidence presented in the literature and then discuss some of the possible interpretations.

Serotonin depletors and neurotoxins

An early hypothesis is due to Meyerson (1964*a,b*), who suggested that 5-HT pathways had an inhibitory effect on oestrus in the rat, and that hormones induced the oestrous state by reducing activity in these 5-HT neurones. He worked with the general neuro-transmitter depleting agent, reserpine, and showed that it could cause enhanced lordosis, which indicates an increase in sexual receptivity. This behaviour appeared to depend on 5-HT, since the admin-istration of its metabolic precursor 5-hydroxytryptophan could reverse the effect of reserpine.

As is the case for the male animal, so there is a large body of work dealing with the effect of PCPA treatment of the female, some of which dates back to the start of the last decade. A good deal of discussion has been provoked by the seemingly contradictory findings of various workers, some of whom find stimulatory effects on lordosis (e.g. Meyerson and Lewander 1970; Ahlenius *et al.* 1972; Zemlan, Ward, Crowley, and Margules 1973; Everitt, Fuxe, and Hökfelt 1974; Everitt, Fuxe, Hökfelt, and Jonsson 1975*a*; Everitt, Fuxe, and Jonsson 1975*a*) while others either claim it has inhibitory effects or even no effects at all (e.g. Sheard 1969; Segal and Whalen 1970; Singer 1972; Eriksson and Södersten 1973; Gorzalka and Whalen 1975; Södersten *et al.* 1976*b*; Al Satli and Aron 1981). However, male patterns of sexual behaviour in the female seem to be reliably enhanced by PCPA (Sheard 1969; Singer 1972; Södersten *et al.* 1976*b*; van de Poll, van Dis, and Bermond 1977).

The effects of *p*-chloramphetamine (pCA) on female receptivity are also debated. The initial action of pCA is to release serotonin from vesicles and to inhibit its reuptake into the terminal, while in the longer term, pCA depletes 5-HT stores in the terminals and causes some neuronal damage. Some workers have reported biphasic behavioural actions that would be in line with these neurochemical effects: suppression of lordosis initially, followed by a prolonged phase of enhanced mating (Zemlan, Trulson, Howell, and Hoebel 1977; Zemlan 1978). However, Södersten *et al.* (1978) could find no effects on lordosis, regardless of whether the animals were progesterone-treated or not, even after oestradiol priming, and quote a variety of reports in support of their assertion that 'drugs affecting 5-HT neurotransmission cannot replace the behavioural effects of [oestradiol] or [progesterone] in ovariectomized rats'.

The drug α-propyldopacetamide blocks 5-HT synthesis without affecting release and also fails to affect female sexual behaviour according to one report (Meyerson and Lewander 1970). Yet Everitt *et al.* (1975*a*) found that it had a stimulatory effect on lordosis similar to that of PCPA, at least when testing was carried out about 2 h after treatment. Unfortunately the longer-term effects are not reported, and in any case this substance is an inhibitor of several enzymes involved in catecholamine metabolism (Carlsson, Corrodi, and Waldeck 1963), so that it is hard to be certain that inhibition of serotonin synthesis was in fact responsible.

Apart from the fact that several of these studies differ from one another with regard to dose, time-course of effects, etc., there is also the problem of interference from non-serotonergic sources. Thus Ahlenius *et al.* (1972), who it will be recalled found that PCPA did enhance lordosis, nevertheless drew attention to the finding that α-methyl-*p*-tyrosine, which acts on the catecholaminergic system, had the same effects as PCPA. They concluded that their data pointed more to control of lordosis by catecholamines than by serotonin.

The oestrous cycle

Perhaps the studies reported by Al Satli (1978; Al Satli and Aron 1981) are also of value here. They are rare in that they deal with serotonin in the intact female in the course of her natural 4-day oestrous cycle, and they provide clear evidence that 5-HT can have opposite effects at different stages in the cycle. Thus a single dose of PCPA given late in the afternoon of diestrus II will inhibit receptivity during the night following proestrus, and this effect can be counteracted by 5-HTP (Al Satli and Aron 1981). Conversely, receptivity can also be reduced by raising 5-HT on the afternoon of proestrus (Al Satli 1978). They conclude '. . . it is reasonable to assume that PCPA suppressed some facilitatory action of 5-HT on the neural structures sensitive to the positive feed-back effects of oestrogens.' Admittedly, it is rather harder to relate these results to ovariectomized females, but it does appear that 5-HT can either enhance or diminish receptivity according to the internal milieu of the animal.

Toxin lesions

Toxin lesions have been investigated by Everitt *et al.* (1975*b*). The serotonergic input to the anterior hypothalamus was selectively abolished by the injection of 5,7-dihydroxytryptamine into the ascending pathway from the raphe nuclei. Lesions were verified 14 days after surgery according to two criteria: firstly, that the high-affinity re-uptake of 5-HT in the hypothalamus was severely reduced, but secondly that there were no effects on noradrenaline re-uptake. This indicates that there was severe and specific destruction of the serotonergic terminals in one target area. During the first week of post-operative testing, the lesioned females showed signs of increasing sexual receptivity, and this effect was very marked from day 6 onwards. However, the effects persisted for at least 150 days thereafter, which we feel raises some doubts about exactly what had been destroyed. Data from our own laboratory show that serotonergic neurones in the hypothalamus are fully restored in females 8 weeks after 5,7-dihydroxytryptamine lesions have been made in the amygdala (File, James, MacLeod, and Wilson, unpublished); and that 5-HT and 5-HIAA levels are no longer significantly reduced 4 weeks after pre-optic area lesions with the same toxin in the male (File, James, and Wilson, unpublished).

While there are therefore regional differences in the rates of regeneration after toxin lesions of the serotonergic systems, it seems that regeneration in the hypothalamus tends to be fast rather than slow. It is therefore regrettable that Everitt *et al.* did not verify their lesions again at the end of behavioural testing.

Central injection of the neurotoxins 5,6- and 5,7-dihydroxy tryptamine was found to elicit mounting behaviour in female rats (DaPrada, Pieri, Keller, Pieri, and Bonetti 1978), again supporting the idea that male patterns of behaviour are under the control of 5-HT, regardless of the sex of the animal. In a similar fashion, Södersten *et al.* (1978) found an increase in the frequency with which the receptive probe females were mounted by the females treated with 5,7-dihydroxytryptamine and by those treated with pCA. This is in full agreement with their earlier data (Södersten *et al.* 1976*b*) regarding PCPA, in which the females even showed behavioural patterns that closely resembled ejaculation, i.e. the deep intromission and slow dismount. (However, the 'refractory period' in the female rat is very much shorter than the true refractory period of the male.) They comment that the data now 'argue against a role of 5-HT in the neural control of lordosis behaviour', but that the full repertoire of male behaviours appears to be latent in the female (Södersten *et al.* 1978).

Receptor antagonists

However, evidence in support of the hypothesis that a reduction in 5-HT transmission does enhance female sexual behaviour, comes from the increased receptivity that followed hypothalamic implantation of the 5-HT receptor antagonist cinanserin (Ward, Crowley, Zemlan, and Margules 1975). Data provided by other workers are also in support of a sexually enhancing effect of receptor-blocking agents. Zemlan *et al.* (1973) introduced both methysergide and cinanserin into the brains of their females and observed increased receptivity, as did Franck and Ward (1981).

Systemic administration can have the same effects, although the picture is more complex; Everitt *et al.* (1975*a*) failed to obtain any effects on behaviour with cinanserin, a potent blocker when applied direct to the brain or studied *in vitro* but with more doubtful effects when applied systemically (Fuxe, unpublished data, cited in Everitt *et al.* 1975*a*). Yet in Hunter and Wilson's hands, cinanserin (10 mg/kg i.p.) was able to further enhance receptivity in oestrogen-treated females (personal communication). The receptor blocker methysergide was studied by Davis and Kohl (1978). Females were ovariectomized and maintained with oestradiol in the usual fashion. A single dose of methysergide induced the behavioural signs of oestrus, as has also been reported by Zemlan *et al.* (1973) and by Henrik and Gerall (1976). However, repeating the dose on subsequent days led to decreasing effects, indicating that some form of compensatory change was occurring. This same phenomenon of behavioural tolerance to treatments which enhance receptivity has also been recorded in experiments with progesterone (Rodriguez-Sierra and Davis 1979).

It was therefore of interest to see whether methysergide and progesterone show cross-tolerance. For this experiment, animals were chronically treated with methysergide and then tested with progesterone present also. Although one would have expected marked tolerance to methysergide after this procedure, progesterone still had as much effect as in the controls, indicating that the mechanisms of stimulation cannot be one and the same. A further dose of progesterone on the following day had a reduced effect, showing that tolerance to the steroid could still occur. Davis and Kohl propose as one explanation of their results that progesterone could be acting via both dopamine and 5-HT. Thus, if the 5-HT circuitry had become tolerant to suppression, as a result of repeated exposure to a receptor blocker, progesterone could nonetheless still induce receptivity by suppressing the dopaminergic neurones. Conversely, if the dopaminergic system was tolerant to the action of progesterone, the steroid could still act via 5-HT suppression. This hypothesis clearly requires further investigation.

Agonists, re-uptake inhibitors, and releasing agents

The raising of 5-HT levels in the brain, which can be accomplished by the concurrent administration of 5-HTP and a monoamine oxidase inhibitor to block its degradation, was reported to inhibit hormonally-induced sexual receptivity (Meyerson 1964*b*). Other manipulations designed to prolong the action of 5-HT, for instance the use of uptake blockers or the facilitation of release by using fenfluramine, also inhibit hormonally-mediated receptivity according to some reports (Everitt *et al.* 1975*a*), although other results are in the opposite direction.

A range of putative serotonergic agonists were selected by Everitt and Fuxe (1977) and tested both for their ability to produce a behavioural syndrome thought to be typical of 5-HT activity, and for their ability to facilitate receptivity. As is generally the case for work on sexual behaviour, the females used were ovariectomized, but for this experiment they were maintained on only a low dose of oestradiol so as to make any enhancement of behaviour more clearly visible. The drugs used were LSD, psilocybin, 5-methoxy dimethyltryptamine, and 3,5-dimethoxy-4-methyl phenylethylamine. In all four cases low doses of the drug enhanced receptivity whereas higher doses had the opposite effect; however, inhibition of lordosis would presumably have been difficult to observe in these rats since the dose of oestradiol used did not induce receptivity by itself. The authors favour the view that this biphasic response reflects stimulation of inhibitory pre-synaptic autoreceptors when the drug is present at low doses, leading to an overall decrease in serotonergic activity, whereas at higher doses there would be a direct effect on the post-synaptic receptors. Thus the results of an overall increase in the activity of the pre-synaptic cell would be mimicked, and this phenomenon has already been referred to in the section on the effects of agonists in the male. However, other explanations are also possible and one will be discussed below.

The paper from Hamburger-Bar *et al.* (1978), cited in the discussion of male behaviour, also considers the effects of these inhibitors in female animals. As far as the female is concerned, ORG 6582, femoxetine, and the rather less specific drug clomipramine, all proved capable of enhancing lordosis behaviour in the presence of progesterone. When tested in the absence of administered progesterone, and in adrenalectomized females, ORG 6582 was still effective, indicating that the effects seen were not due to the release of progesterone from the adrenals. The authors state, in their discussion of the conflicting results that have been obtained from work with PCPA, that 'the results for the 5-HT reuptake inhibitors (suggest) that the influence of 5-HT on the regulation of lordosis is not solely an inhibitory one'.

Effects of zimelidine

Hunter and Wilson (1982) have used the 5-HT re-uptake inhibitors zimelidine, and Wy 26002, employing two different doses of oestrogen. On dividing their results according to presence or absence of female receptivity, they found that zimelidine would inhibit the lordotic response in otherwise receptive animals. These data are supported by work reported by Everitt *et al.* (1975*a*), who describe results obtained with fenfluramine, a drug which initially causes release of serotonin (followed later by some depletion). This substance decreased receptivity about 1 h after injection, although the sedative effects of fenfluramine might account for that action. Zimelidine, however, would actually facilitate the behaviour in Hunter and Wilson's previously non-responding animals. Unfortunately, they did not carry out the logical follow-up to these experiments, namely to treat the previously unreceptive females with zimelidine for a second time, in order to discover whether they differed in any way from those females that were receptive from the first. However, it could be argued that the effects of that type of sub-chronic administration might be a complicating factor.

If zimelidine were a pure 5-HT re-uptake inhibitor, one would be tempted to conclude that raising the level of 5-HT can induce some plastic change in the relevant neural circuitry, and that subsequent pulses of 5-HT are then inhibitory. Unfortunately, though, zimelidine *in vivo* is as potent as inhibitor of noradrenaline reuptake as of serotonin (Moser, Wood, and Wyllie 1981). The results from the Wy 26002 compound, which appears to be as selective for 5-HT *in vivo* as it is *in vitro*, reveal no inhibitory effects. In fact, some of the receptive females showed even higher lordosis quotients when tested with this drug. In any event it seems clear that raising the levels of 5-HT is certainly one way of stimulating the lordotic response.

Possible mechanisms

As was suggested at the beginning of this chapter, the role of 5-HT in the control of female receptivity is very much less well understood than its role in the male. It should be apparent that both PCPA and re-uptake inhibitors seem to produce opposite effects in the hands of different workers. For instance, acute treatment with PCPA will enhance receptivity in ovariectomized females treated with oestradiol. However, in the majority of cases this effect has only been seen a few hours after injection, at a time when the biochemical picture is one of 5-HT release and NA depletion rather than specific 5-HT depletion. It is therefore less surprising to note that chronic treatment (Segal and Whalen 1970), or even a single dose given 24 h before oestrogen-priming of the animal (Gorzalka and Whalen 1975), is ineffective and can indeed impair the ability of progesterone to produce receptivity. These treatments would be expected to cause the depletion of 5-HT to be more specific, and chronic treatment especially so. Results with other depletors are also complicated by problems of time-course, specificity, and so on.

A recent paper investigates several details of the actions of PCPA, using ovariectomized, oestradiol-maintained females, and does a good deal to clarify the problems involved when this drug is used (Wilson *et al.* 1982). First, the dose–response relationship was established for the acute effects of PCPA metabolite *p*-chlorophenylethylamine (PCPEA). An increased lordosis quotient resulted from all doses of PCPA, but the effect of 150 mg/kg was significantly greater than of 100, 200, or 300 mg/kg. Furthermore, the dose–response curves for the effects on receptivity and the effects on indoleamines were far from parallel; even more striking was the finding that the precursor 5-HTP was able to maintain 5-HIAA levels, and in fact to raise 5-HT, without affecting the behaviour. The i.c.v. administration of noradrenaline reduced receptivity at a dose that did not affect motor activity in general, and was also capable of reducing the receptivity of female rats treated with progesterone rather than PCPA. Conversely, a 30day course of PCPA (150 mg kg^{-1} day^{-1}) had no effect on lordosis, despite a fall in 5-HT levels to some 25 per cent of control and the loss of 5-HIAA to below the detection limit of the assay; catecholamine levels were not affected.

The decarboxylated PCPA metabolite *p*-chlorophenylethylamine is known to stimulate the efflux of 5-HT from terminals as well as reducing NA content, and it is likely that some of the *in vivo* effects of PCPA in fact result from this metabolite (Sloviter, Drust, and Connor 1978). Wilson, Bonney, Everard, Parrott, and Wise (1982) report that *p*-chlorophenylethylamine (20 mg/kg) stimulated lordosis 1 h after injection, but with a bimodal effect: some animals became highly receptive whilst others were unaffected. Both hypothalamic 5-HT and NA were reduced by this treatment. When the decarboxylase inhibitor benserazide was used, subsequent administration of PCPA led to less stimulation than was observed in the absence of benserazide, and in the group receiving the combination, NA was unchanged while 5-HIAA was reduced. Thus at least some of the PCPA effect may be due to the 5-HT release occasioned by the metabolite, which would of course match well with the data obtained from work with re-uptake inhibitors and low doses of agonists, but is harder to reconcile with the data from antagonists and higher doses of agonists.

Two final experiments were concerned with the interaction between 5-HT and progesterone. First, PCPA was shown to stimulate adrenal steroidogenesis, leading to a 50 per cent increase in the plasma progesterone concentration 4 h later. Secondly, progesterone, when injected subcutaneously, caused a decrease in 5-HT in the hypothalamus whilst 5-HIAA was maintained, this being an indication that 5-HT release was stimulated by the steroid.

In conclusion, then, the effects of PCPA might result from one or more of the following three actions. Adrenal progesterone output is enhanced, and this will in turn strengthen the effect of injected hormone, or add to that re-leased following a natural LH surge. PCPA rapidly depletes NA by stimulating its efflux from stores in the terminals, and it seems likely that NA may exert an inhibitory action on receptivity (it is interesting to speculate on the involve-ment of noradrenaline in the results reported for zimelidine above). PCPEA both depletes NA and causes a transient burst of 5-HT release.

We shall confine ourselves to discussion of the last-mentioned possibility, since it allows some interpretation of other data. The biphasic effects of agonist drugs have already been mentioned; it is perhaps tempting to consider that a low dose of agonist would have the same effects as the transient pulse of serotonin. The inhibition of behaviour that results from higher doses might then be due to a desensitization phenomenon rather than differential activation of auto- and post-synaptic receptors. It will require work with more highly receptor-selective compounds than are currently available before this question can be resolved. However, it is known that chronic treatment with progesterone ceases to activate and actually inhibits receptivity (Rodriguez-Sierra and Davis 1979), an effect which could equally well be due to exhaustion of the pre-synaptic stores of transmitter, or to receptor desensitization.

Pre-depletion of 5-HT will block the action of progesterone (Segal and Whalen, *op. cit.*), and the 'clean' tryptophan hydroxylase inhibitor α-propyl-dopacetamide, which blocks 5-HT synthesis without affecting release, also fails to affect female sexual behaviour (Meyerson and Lewander 1970). As for the data from fenfluramine, it would seem necessary to invoke some form of 'overload inhibition' (resulting from the prolonged presence of high levels of 5-HT at the receptors) if one wished to save the transient release theory. Of course, this might be precisely the manner by which an initial dose of progesterone can diminish the effects of later ones, as discussed by Davis and Kohl (1978).

CONCLUSIONS

It is now very well established that male patterns of sexual behaviour are en-hanced in both males and females by treatments that lower brain 5-HT and are inhibited by those that increase 5-HT levels. What is not yet so clear is the extent to which the animals will respond again and again to alterations in sero-tonin and to what extent changes in performance tend to persist after the serotonin levels have returned to their pre-challenge values.

With regard to female patterns, it seems hard to draw firm conclusions at present. It is argued by some that serotonin is not involved in lordosis; however, we find this statement too strong. The next year or so should produce further work clarifying the opposing effects that some drugs seem to exert. It is tempting to speculate that the serotonergic cells with their bodies in the ventro-medial nucleus may have been responsible for some of the complex effects that have been observed, since their responses to serotonergic manipulations may be quite different to responses of other cells. Besides, the complex spectra of action of the drugs available for manipulating 5-HT make all conclusions rather tentative.

We conclude with a brief look at the effects of serotonergic drugs on human sexual response. There appear to be extremely little data on this subject; the few effectors of the 5-HT systems which are available tend not to be widely used (with the exception of anti-depressants of course), perhaps because of their unpleasant side-effects. We simply cannot say to what extent the results from the rat can be extrapolated to the clinic; yet the changes in libido and response that may result from drug treatment can have intense personal significance for the patient.

Eaton (1973) reports the use of clomipramine in the treatment of premature ejaculation, which would fit in well with the concept that raised 5-HT levels cause some inhibition of response, and especially with the data from Ahlenius *et al.* (1979) that has been quoted above. More recently, Goodman (1980) reported on a double-blind cross-over trial with clomipramine in men suffering from premature ejaculation. The drug proved moderately successful, although the well-documented side-effects of the tricyclics that result from their blockade of histamine and acetylcholine receptors (e.g. dry mouth, constipation, drowsiness) did cause some discomfort. Goodman suggests that the underlying effect may in fact be reduction of anxiety by the drug.

However, it seems that the 'aphrodisiac' effects (Gessa *et al.* 1971) of PCPA that are so clear in the male rat fail to appear in man. In early work on the compound, Cremata and Koe (1966, 1968), observed no change in the sexual behaviour of a sample of prison inmates, and Sjoerdsma *et al.* (1970), in reviewing 16 cases, also reported no evidence of changed self-ratings for sexual interest. What was reported were the following effects: 'fatigue, dizziness, nausea, uneasiness and headache' (Cremata and Koe 1966) and 'restlessness, anxiety, agitation, crying and depression' (Sjoerdsma *et al.* 1970). However, combined PCPA and testosterone treatment of patients who complained of migraine and sexual dysfunction did prove effective, as measured by the incidence of erections stimulated by erotic imagery (Sicuteri 1974). One wonders, though, whether this was not more the result of the testosterone than the PCPA itself.

Perhaps the biggest drawback is that all these serotonergic drugs also have peripheral actions which can interfere with their intended effects. For instance, the 5-HT antagonist methysergide apparently causes drowsiness, confusion, insomnia, nausea, and diarrhoea, although the drug has also been used to control diarrhoea resulting from carcinoid syndrome or from fenfluramine medication (Kruk and Pycock 1979). It seems clear that serotonergic effectors are not very promising as aphrodisiacs.

References

Aghajanian, G. K., Haigler, H. G., and Bennett, J. L. (1975). Amine receptors in CNS. III: 5-hydroxytryptamine in brain. In *Handbook of psychopharmacology*, vol. 6; *Biogenic amine Receptors* (eds. Iversen, L. L., Iversen, S. D., and Snyder, S. H.) pp. 63–96. Plenum Press, New York.

Ahlenius, S., Engel, J., Eriksson, H., Modigh, K., and Södersten, P. (1972). Importance of central catecholamines in the mediation of lordosis behaviour in ovariectomised rats treated with oestrogen and inhibitors of monoamine synthesis. *J. Neural Trans.* **33**, 247–55.

—— Heimann, M., and Larsson, K. (1979). Prolongation of the ejaculation latency in the male rat by thioridazine and chlorimipramine. *Psychopharmacology* **65**, 137–40.

—— Larsson, K., and Svensson, L. (1980*a*). Stimulating effects of lisuride on masculine sexual behavior of rats. *Eur. J. Pharmac.* **64**, 47–51.

—— —— —— (1980*b*). Further evidence for an inhibitory role of central 5-HT in male rat sexual behavior. *Psychopharmacology* **68**, 217–20.

—— —— —— Hjorth, S., Carlsson, A., Lindberg, P., Wikström, H., Sanchez, D., Arvidsson, L. -E., Hacksell, U., and Nilsson, J. L. G. (1981). Effects of a new type of 5-HT receptor agonist on male rat sexual behavior. *Pharmac. Biochem. Behav.* **15**, 785–92.

Al Satli, M. (1978). Données nouvelles sur le controle serotonergique de la receptivité sexuelle chez la ratte. *C. r. Hebd. Seanc. Acad. Sci. Paris* **286**, 1253–5.

—— and Aron, C. (1981). Role played by serotonin in the control of estrous receptivity, ovarian activity and ovulation in the cyclic female rat. *Psychoneuroendocrinology* **6**, 121–9.

Azmitia, E. C. and Segal, M. (1978). An autoradiographic analysis of the differential ascending projections of the dorsal and median raphe nuclei in the rat. *J. Comp. Neurol.* **179**, 641–68.

Barfield, R. J. and Chen, J. J. (1977). Activation of estrous behavior in ovariectomised rats by intra-cerebral implants of estradiol benzoate. *Endocrinology* **101**, 1716–25.

Barfield, R. J. and Geyer, L. (1975). The ultra-sonic post-ejaculatory vocalization and the post-ejaculatory refractory period in the male rat. *J. Comp. Physiol. Psychol.* **88**, 723–34.

Baum, M. J. and Starr, M. S. (1980). Inhibition of sexual behavior by dopamine antagonist or serotonin agonist drugs in castrated male rats given estradiol or dihydrotestosterone. *Pharmac. Biochem. Behav.* **13**, 57–67.

Benkert, O. and Eversmann, T. (1972). Importance of the anti-serotonin effect for mounting behaviour in male rats. *Experientia* **28**, 532–3.

Bond, V. J., Shillito, E. E., and Vogt, M. (1972). Influence of age and of testosterone on the response of male rats to *p*-chlorophenylalanine. *Br. J. Pharmac.* **46**, 46–55.

Carlsson, A., Corrodi, H., and Waldeck, B. (1963). α-Substituierte Dopacetamide als Hemmer der Catechol-*o*-methyltransferase und der enzymatischen Hydroxylierung aromatischer Aminosäuren: in den Catecholamine-Metabolismus eingreifende Substanzen. *Helv. Chim. Acta* **46**, 2271–86.

Chan-Palay, V. (1977). Indoleamine neurons and their processes in the normal rat brain and in chronic diet-induced thiamin deficiency, demonstrated by uptake of [^{3}H]-serotonin. *J. Comp. Neurol.* **176**, 467–94.

Christensen, L. W. and Clemens, L. G. (1975). Blockade of testosterone-induced mounting behaviour in the male rat with intracranial application of the aromatization inhibitor androst-1,4,6-triene-3,17-dione. *Endocrinology* **97**, 1545–51.

Cremata, V. Y. and Koe, B. K. (1966). Clinical-pharmacological evaluation of p-chlorophenylalanine: a new serotonin-depleting agent. Clin. Pharmacol. Ther. 7, 768-76.
—— —— (1968). Clinical and biochemical effects of fenclonine, a serotonin depletor. Dis. Nerv. Syst. 29, 147-52.
Crowley, W. R., Ward, I. L., and Margules, D. L. (1975). Female lordotic behaviour mediated by monoamines in male rats. J. Comp. Physiol. Psychol. 88, 62-8.
Dahlström, A. and Fuxe, K. (1964). Evidence for the existence of monoamine-containing neurons in the CNS. I: Demonstration of monoamines in the cell bodies of brain stem neurons. Acta Physiol. Scand. Suppl. 232, 1-55.
Da Prada, M., Carruba, M., O'Brien, R., Saner, A., and Pletscher, A. (1972). The effect of 5,6-dihydroxytryptamine on sexual behaviour of male rats. Eur. J. Pharmac. 79, 288-90.
—— Bonetti, E. P., and Keller, H. H. (1977). Induction of mounting behavior in female and male rats by lisuride. Neurosci. Lett. 6, 349-53.
—— Pieri, L., Keller, H. H., Pieri, M., and Bonetti, E. P. (1978). Effects of 5,6-dihydroxytryptamine and 5,7-dihydroxytryptamine on the rat central nervous system after intraventricular or intracerebral application and on blood platelets in vivo. Ann. N. Y. Acad. Sci. 305, 595-620.
Davis, G. A. and Kohl, R. L. (1978). Biphasic effects of the anti-serotonergic methysergide on lordosis in rats. Pharmac. Biochem. Behav. 9, 487-91.
del Fiaco, M., Fratta, W., Gessa, G. L., and Tagliamonte, A. (1974). Lack of copulatory behaviour in male castrated rats after p-chlorophenylalanine. Br. J. Pharmac. 51, 249-51.
Eaton, H. (1973). Chlorimipramine (Anafranil) in the treatment of premature ejaculation. J. Int. Med. Res. 1, 432-4.
Eriksson, H. and Södersten, P. (1973). A failure to facilitate lordosis behavior in adrenalectomized and gonadectomized estrogen-primed rats with monoamine synthesis inhibitors. Horm. Behav. 4, 89-97.
Everitt, B. J. (1977). Cerebral monoamines and sexual behaviour. In Handbook of sexology (eds. J. Money and H. Musaph). pp. 429-48. Excerpta Medica, Amsterdam.
—— and Fuxe, K. (1977). Serotonin and sexual behavior in female rats. Effects of hallucinogenic indolealkylamines and phenylethylamines. Neurosci. Lett. 4, 215-20.
—— —— and Hökfelt, T. (1974). Inhibitory role of dopamine and 5-hydroxy-tryptamine in the sexual behaviour of female rats. Eur. J. Pharmacol. 29, 187-91.
—— —— —— and Jonsson, G. (1975). Role of monoamines in the control of sexual receptivity in the female rat. J. Comp. Physiol. Psychol. 89, 556-72.
—— —— and Jonsson, G. (1975). The effects of 5,7-dihydroxytryptamine lesions of ascending 5-hydroxytryptamine pathways on the sexual and aggressive behaviour of female rats. J. Pharmacol. (Paris) 6, 25-32.
File, S. E. and Wardill, A. (1975). Validity of head-dipping as a measure of exploration in a modified hole-board. Psychopharmacologia 44, 53-9.
—— and Tucker, J. C. (1983). Neonatal clomipramine in the rat does not affect social, sexual and exploratory behaviors in adulthood. Neurobehav. Toxicol. Teratol. 5, 3-8.
—— James, T. A. and MacLeod, N. K. (1981). Depletion in amygdaloid 5-hydroxy-tryptamine concentration and changes in social and aggressive behaviour. J. Neural Trans. 50, 1-12.
Franck, J. E. and Ward, I. L. (1981). Intralimbic progesterone and methysergide facilitate lordotic behavior in estrogen-primed female rats. Neuroendocrinology 32, 50-6.
Gessa, G. L., Tagliamonte, A., and Tagliamonte, P. (1971). Aphrodisiac effect

of *p*-chlorophenylalanine. *Science* **171**, 706.

—— —— —— and Brodie, B. B. (1970). Essential role of testosterone in the sexual stimulation induced by *p*-chlorophenylalanine in male animals. *Nature, Lond.* **227**, 616–17.

Ginton, A. (1976). Copulation in non-copulators: effect of PCPA in male rats. *Pharmac. Biochem. Behav.* **4**, 357–9.

Goodman, R. E. (1980). An assessment of clomipramine (Anafranil) in the treatment of premature ejaculation. *J. Int. Med. Res.* **8**, Suppl. 3: 53–9.

Gorzalka, B. B. and Whalen, R. E. (1975). Inhibition, not facilitation, of sexual behavior by PCPA. *Pharmac. Biochem. Behav.* **3**, 511–13.

Grant, L. D. and Stumpf, W. E. (1976). Hormone uptake sites in relation to CNS biogenic amine systems. In *Anatomical neuroendocrinology* (eds. W. E. Stumpf and L. D. Grant) pp. 445–63. Karger, New York.

Hamburger-Bar, R., Rigter, H., and Dekker, I. (1978). Inhibition of serotonin reuptake differentially affects heterosexual behavior of male and female rats. *Life Sci.* **22**, 1827–36.

Heimer, L. and Larsson, K. (1966). Impairment of mating behaviour in male rats following lesions in the preoptic-anterior hypothalamic continuum. *Brain Res.* **3**, 248–63.

Henrik, E. and Gerall, A. A. (1976). Facilitation of receptivity in estrogen-primed rats during successive mating tests with progestins and methysergide. *J. Comp. Physiol. Psychol.* **90**, 590–600.

Hunter, J. A. and Wilson, C. A. (1982). The stimulatory effects of 5-HT on female sexual behaviour. Abstract in *4th Conference of European Society for Comparative Physiology and Biochemistry*. Liège, Belgium. Eur. Soc. Comp. Physiol. Biochem. (ed. J. Balthazart) pp. 234–5.

Krieger, M. S., Orr, D., and Perper, T. (1976). Temporal patterning of sexual behavior in the female rat. *Behav. Biol.* **18**, 379–86.

Kruk, Z. L. and Pycock, C. J. (1979). *Neurotransmitters and drugs*, p. 102. Croom-Helm, London.

Larsson, K. and Södersten, P. (1971). Lordosis behavior in male rats treated with estrogen in combination with tetrabenazine and nialamide. *Psychophysiology* **21**, 13–16.

—— Fuxe, K., Everitt, B. J., Holmgren, M., and Södersten, P. (1978). Sexual behavior in male rats after intracerebral injection of 5,7-dihydroxytryptamine. *Brain Res.* **141**, 293–303.

Leedy, M. G., Vela, E. A., Popolow, H. B., and Gerall, A. A. (1980). Effect of prepubertal medial preoptic area lesions on male rat sexual behavior. *Physiol. Behav.* **24**, 341–6.

Malmnäs, C. O. (1973). Monoaminergic influences on testosterone-activated copulatory behaviour in the castrated male rat. *Acta Physiol. Scand. Suppl.* **395**, 1–128.

—— and Meyerson, B. J. (1971). *p*-Chlorophenylalanine and copulatory behaviour in the male rat. *Nature, Lond.* **232**, 394–400.

Malsbury, C. W. (1971). Facilitation of male rat copulatory behaviour by electrical stimulation of the medial pre-optic area. *Physiol. Behav.* **7**, 795–805.

Mathews, K. and Edwards, A. (1977). Involvement of ventromedial and anterior hypothalamic nuclei in the hormonal induction of receptivity in the female rat. *Physiol. Behav.* **19**, 319–26.

McClintock, M. (1974). Sociobiology of reproduction in the Norway rat (*Rattus norvegicus*): estrous synchrony and the role of the female rat in copulatory behavior. Unpublished doctoral thesis, Department of Psychology, University of Pennsylvania.

McIntosh, T. K., Davis, P. G., and Barfield, R. J. (1979). Urine marking and sexual behavior in the rat (*Rattus norvegicus*). *Behav. Neural Biol.* **26**, 161–8.

Meyerson, B. J. (1964*a*). The effect of neuropharmacological agents on hormone-activated oestrous behaviour in ovariectomised rats. *Arch. Int. Pharmacodyn. Ther.* **150**, 4–33.

—— (1964*b*). Central nervous monoamines and hormone-induced oestrous behaviour in the spayed rat. *Acta Physiol. Scand. Suppl.* **241**, 1–31.

—— (1968). Female copulatory behaviour in male and androgenised female rats after oestrogen/amine depletor treatment. *Nature, Lond.* **217**, 683.

—— and Lewander, T. (1970). Serotonin synthesis inhibition and estrous behavior in female rats. *Life Sci.* **9**, 661–71.

Mirmiran, M., van de Poll, N., Corner, M., van Oyen, H., and Bour, H. (1981). Suppression of active sleep by chronic treatment with chlorimipramine during early postnatal development: effects upon adult sleep and behavior in the rat. *Brain Res.* **204**, 129–46.

Mitler, M., Morden, B., Levine, S., and Dement, W. (1972). The effects of *p*-chlorophenylalanine on the mating behavior of male rats. *Physiol. Behav.* **8**, 1147–50.

Morden, B., Mullins, S., Levine, S., Cohen, H., and Dement, W. (1968). Effect of REM sleep deprivation on the mating behavior of male rats. *Psychophysiology* **5**, 241–2.

Moser, P. C., Wood, M. D., and Wyllie, M. G. (1981). Selective inhibition of 5-HT uptake *in vivo. Br. J. Pharmac.* **74**, 888P.

Nance, D. W., Christensen, L. W., Shryne, J. E., and Gorski, R. A. (1977). Modifications in gonadotropin control and reproductive behavior in the female rat by hypothalamic and pre-optic lesions. *Brain Res. Bull.* **2**, 307–12.

Pfaff, D. W. and Sakuma, Y. (1979*a*). Facilitation of the lordosis reflex of female rats from the ventromedial nucleus of the hypothalamus. *J. Physiol.* **288**, 189–202.

—— —— (1979*b*). Deficit in the lordosis reflex of female rats caused by lesions in the ventromedial nucleus of the hypothalamus. *J. Physiol.* **288**, 203–10.

Powers, B. and Valenstein, E. S. (1972). Sexual receptivity: facilitation by medial pre-optic lesions in female rats. *Science* **175**, 1003–5.

Raisman, G. and Field, P. M. (1973). Sexual dimorphism in the neuropil of the preoptic area of the rat and its dependence on neonatal androgen. *Brain Res.* **54**, 1–29.

Rodriguez-Sierra, J. F. and Davis, G. A. (1979). Tolerance to the lordosis-facilitatory effects of progesterone or methysergide. *Neuropharmacology* **18**, 335–9.

Rogawski, M. A. and Aghajanian, G. K. (1978). Response of central monoaminergic neurons to lisuride: comparison with LSD. *Life Sci.* **24**, 1289–98.

Salis, P. G. and Dewsbury, D. A. (1971). *p*-Chlorophenylalanine stimulates copulatory behaviour in male rats. *Nature, Lond.* **232**, 400–1.

Segal, D. S. and Whalen, R. E. (1970). Effect of chronic administration of *p*-chlorophenylalanine on sexual receptivity of the female rat. *Psychopharmacologia* **16**, 434–8.

Sheard, M. H. (1969). The effects of *p*-chlorophenylalanine on behaviour in rats: relation to brain serotonin and 5-hydroxyindole acetic acid. *Brain Res.* **15**, 524–8.

Shillito, E. (1969). The effect of *p*-chlorophenylalanine on social interactions of male rats. *Br. J. Pharmac.* **36**, 193–4P.

—— (1970). The effect of *p*-chlorophenylalanine on social interaction of male rats. *Br. J. Pharmac.* **38**, 305–15.

—— and Vogt, M. (1978). Excessive social and sexual interactions in rats: relation to changes in brain amines. *Neuroscience* **3**, 241–9.

Sicuteri, F. (1974). Serotonin and sex in man. *Pharmac. Res. Commun.* **6**, 403–11.

Singer, J. J. (1972). Effects of *p*-chlorophenylalanine on the male and female sexual behaviour of female rats. *Psychol. Rep.* **30**, 891–3.

Sjoerdsma, A., Lovenberg, W., Engelman, K., Carpenter, W. T., Wyatt, R. J., and Gessa, G. L. (1970). Serotonin now: clinical implications of inhibiting its synthesis with *p*-chlorophenylalanine. *Ann. Int. Med.* **73**, 607–29.

Sloviter, R. S., Drust, E. G., and Connor, J. D. (1978). Serotonin agonist actions of *p*-chlorophenylalanine. *Neuropharmacology* **17**, 1029–33.

Södersten, P. and Ahlenius, S. (1972). Female lordosis behavior in oestrogen-primed male rats treated with *p*-chlorophenylalanine or *a*-methyl-*p*-tyrosine. *Horm. Behav.* **3**, 181–9.

—— Berge, O. G., and Hole, K. (1978). Effects of *p*-chloroamphetamine and 5,7-dihydroxy tryptamine on the sexual behavior of gonadectomized male and female rats. *Pharmac. Biochem. Behav.* **9**, 499–508.

—— Larsson, K., Ahlenius, S., and Engel, J. (1976*a*). Sexual behavior in castrated male rats treated with monoamine synthesis inhibitors and testosterone. *Pharmac. Biochem. Behav.* **5**, 319–27.

—— —— —— —— (1976*b*). Stimulation of mounting behavior but not lordosis behavior in ovariectomised female rats by *p*-chlorophenylalanine. *Pharmac. Biochem. Behav.* **5**, 329–33.

Stevens, D. A. and Koster, E. P. (1972). Open field responses of rats to stressed and unstressed predecessor urine. *Behav. Biol.* **7**, 519–25.

Tagliamonte, A., Tagliamonte, P., Gessa, G. L. and Brodie, B. B. (1969). Compulsive sexual activity induced by *p*-chlorophenylalanine in normal and pinealectomised male rats. *Science* **166**, 1433–5.

—— —— Stern, S., and Gessa, G. L. (1970). Inhibition of sexual behavior in male rats by a monoamine oxidase inhibitor (MAOI), reversal of this effect by *p*-chlorophenylalanine (PCPA). *Clin. Res.* **18**, 671.

Thor, D. H. and Holloway, W. R. (1981). Persistence of social investigatory behavior in the male rat: evidence for long-term memory of initial copulatory experience. *Anim. Learn. Behav.* **9**, 561–5.

van de Kar, L. D. and Lorens, S. A. (1979). Differential serotonergic innervation of individual hypothalamic nuclei and other forebrain regions by the dorsal and median midbrain raphe nuclei. *Brain Res.* **162**, 45–54.

van de Poll, N. E., van Dis, H., and Bermond, B. (1977). The induction of mounting behavior in female rats by *p*-chlorophenylalanine. *Eur. J. Pharmac.* **41**, 225–9.

van Dis, H. and Larsson, K. (1971). Induction of sexual arousal in the castrated male rat by intracranial stimulation. *Physiol. Behav.* **6**, 85–6.

Ward, I. L., Crowley, W. R., Zemlan, F. P., and Margules, D. L. (1975). Monoaminergic mediation of female sexual behavior. *J. Comp. Physiol. Psychol.* **88**, 53–61.

Whalen, R. E. and Luttge, W. G. (1970). Parachlorophenylalanine methyl ester: an aphrodisiac? *Science* **169**, 1000–1.

Wilson, C. A., Bonney, R. C., Everard, D. M., Parrott, R. F., and Wise, J. (1982). Mechanisms of action of *p*-chlorophenylalanine in stimulating sexual receptivity in the female rat. *Pharmac. Biochem. Behav.* **16**, 777–84.

Yamanouchi, K. (1980). Inhibitory and facilitatory neural mechanisms involved in the regulation of lordosis behavior in female rats: effects of dual cuts in the pre-optic area and hypothalamus. *Physiol. Behav.* **25**, 721–5.

Zemlan, F. P. (1978). Influence of *p*-chloroamphetamine and *p*-chlorophenyl-alanine on female mating behavior. *Ann. N.Y. Acad. Sci.* **305**, 621–6.

—— Ward, I. L., Crowley, W. R. and Margules, D. L. (1973). Activation of lordotic responding in female rats by suppression of serotonergic activity. *Science* **179**, 1010–11.

—— Trulson, M. E., Howell, R. and Hoebel, B. G. (1977). Influence of *p*-chloroamphetamine on female sexual reflexes and brain monoamine levels. *Br. Res.* **123**, 347–356.

4

Sex hormones and the brain

H. KOPERA

INTRODUCTION

SEX HORMONES, i.e. oestrogens, progestins, and androgens, are substances produced in the organism. However, in therapy and in most experiments, artificial compounds are used which have activities similar to those of sex hormones. Hence in this paper no differentiation will be made between the natural hormones and hormone-like artificial substances. Furthermore, very frequently there is such an inextricable interaction between the hormones, that in many instances effects of any single hormone cannot be distinguished satisfactorily.

The actions of sex hormones are by no means confined to the reproductive organs. On the contrary, their targets are almost all tissues and vital systems.

TABLE 4.1 *Targets of sex hormones*

Central nervous system
Autonomic nervous system
Endocrine organs
Bone, fatty tissue, skin
Vessels, circulation, blood
Water–electrolyte balance
Metabolism, gastric secretion
Urinary tract

Reproductive organs

The action of sex hormones on the brain, the affective state, overt behaviour, and neuroendocrine function is the subject of this brief review, which is an extension of one published earlier (Kopera 1980). For details and exhaustive literature see the following references: Arnold (1980), Bäckström (1977), Dörner (1979), Editorial (1979), Eisenfeld (1972), Herbert (1977), Itil, Laudahn, and Herrmann (1976), Junkmann (1968/69), Kopera (1973), McEwen and Parsons (1982), Porter and Whelan (1979), Sachar (1976), Sawyer (1971), Tausk and de Visser (1971), Vernikos-Danellis (1972), and de Wied and van Keep (1980).

HORMONE DISTRIBUTION

Oestrogens

After injection of labelled oestradiol, radioactivity in all brain regions exceeds blood levels by a factor of 3 or more, but oestrogens are taken up and distributed differentially in various areas of the central nervous system (CNS) (Eisenfeld 1972; Stumpf, Sar, and Keefer 1975). The specific accumulation of oestrogens is greatest in the basal hypothalamus, the preoptic regions, and the amygdala, which all seem to constitute the core of the oestrogen sensory limbic system, and in the anterior pituitary. In rats, 1 h after i.v. administration the concentration of oestrogens in the anterior pituitary is about 100 times greater than in plasma. The hormone is taken up to a greater extent by the neurones. Oestrogens attach to protein-containing macromolecules, and specific nuclear and cytosol receptors have been identified in various areas of the brain including the hypothalamus, the anterior pituitary, and the preoptic area. The anterior pituitary contains a 60-fold, and the hypothalamus at least a 10-fold, higher concentration of specific binding macromolecules than, for example, cerebrum or cerebellum. A potent competition by catechol oestrogen (Fishman 1977) for oestrogen receptors of the pituitary and hypothalamus has been reported, which has been assumed to be of possible physiological significance. The concentration of catechol oestrogens in hypothalamus and pituitary was found to be at least 10 times higher than for the parent oestrogens (Paul and Axelrod 1977).

There is a clear relation between the plasma hormone levels and the levels in the cerebrospinal fluid (CSF). It was reported that the levels in the CSF were in agreement with the calculated unbound, i.e. the physiologically active, oestrogen plasma fraction.

Progesterone

Progesterone also seems to be taken up into the brain rather rapidly. It accumulates more in the midbrain than in the hypothalamus, cerebral cortex, or hippocampus. The rat brain contains one progestin receptor system in the hypothalamus and pre-optic area, which is oestrogen regulated, and another in the midbrain and cerebral cortex, which is insensitive to elevated plasma oestrogen (MacLusky and McEwen 1978). Progesterone has no effect on the hypothalamic oestradiol binding capacity. In contrast to other target organs, uptake of female sex hormones in neural tissues is not influenced by the age of the animal or by the adrenals. However, hormone priming can enhance hormone retention in some brain areas. It is assumed that the effects of progesterone in regulating the timing of ovulation and sexual behaviour of the rat may be related to the effect on oestradiol retention in the CNS (Lisk and Reuter 1977).

Testosterone

Radioactive testosterone is also differentially distributed in the brain of immature rats, with highest concentrations in the olfactory bulbs, spinal cord, and posterior and anterior hypothalamus. Androgen receptors have so far only been detected in adult male and female rats. After administration of labelled testosterone, both testosterone and dihydrotestosterone are found in the hypothalamus and pituitary (Eisenfeld 1972); however, the effect of androgens on sexual behaviour and sex-specific characteristics does not seem to be mediated by 5α-dihydrotestosterone (McDonald, Tan, Beyer, Sampson,

Newton, Kitching, Bresci, Greenhill, Baker, and Pritchard 1970; Whalen and Luttge 1971).

CEREBRAL EFFECTS

Sex hormones exert regulatory influences on the CNS, particularly during limited 'critical' periods in the rapidly developing embryonic, foetal, and postnatal brain. They result in sexual differentiation and profound modification of both sexual and non-sexual behaviour and endocrine function in the adult animal.

Sex differences

Female and male brains differ, amongst other respects, in relation to gonado-trophin regulation and behaviour. Males secrete FSH and LH constantly (tonic secretion), whilst females have a cyclic discharge. Aromatizable androgens are converted during infancy into oestrogens, by central neuroendocrine tissues in localized areas related to reproductive function (Naftolin, Ryan, Davies, Reddy, Flores, Petro, and Kuhn 1975).

Many recent data support the concept that in the period of hypothalamic differentiation, oestrogens are essential for sexual differentiation. This involves both the suppression of the female patterns of gonadotrophin secretion and sexual behaviour, and the central organization of normal patterns of male sexual behaviour (Booth 1978). Thus the oestrogens derived from androgens by intraneuronal conversion may serve as the actual masculinising hormones. This is assumed for rodents; for primates it is uncertain whether androgens exert their masculinizing effect directly or only after conversion to oestrogens (Goy and McEwen 1980). On the other hand, it can also be of great importance that abundantly available α-foetoprotein, which binds oestrogens with extra-ordinarily high affinity but does not bind testosterone, shields the female brain from plasma oestrogens; while the male brain is exposed to testicular androgens and the animal is masculinized.

Oestrogen deficiency

In mammals lack of oestrogens results in a cyclical schedule of gonadotrophin secretion and in female sexual behaviour, unless sufficient androgens are present during early development, because the inherent programme in both sexes is female. The exposure of an undifferentiated brain to sex steroids is a necessary requirement for the development of an acyclic pattern of gonadotrophin se-cretion (Arai 1981). Administration of androgens to females within the first days after birth prevents ovulation at maturity. Neonatally, androgen-treated females possibly do not respond to oestrogens as well as normal females; they show less frequently the behaviour pattern characteristic for oestrogens, i.e. assuming a lordotic position when mounted by a male. Possibly the reduced responsiveness is due to a defective oestrogen binding.

For some species, centres sensitive to the action of sex hormones and respon-sible for the control over sexual behaviour have been located. Presumably they have to be primed prenatally to enable steroids to act on them in the adult animal. The differentiation of such centres seems to depend on the concentrations of the oestrogens rather than the type of the hormone. Pre- and neonatally, oestrogens cause a pronounced proliferation of these hormone-sensitive centres, increasing the number of neurones and dendritic synapses. Sex hormones continue to modify the structure of the hypothalamus until puberty, and in appropriate amounts may even affect the structures in adult life; in the rat persistent oestrus and polycystic ovaries have been shown to be associated with an oestrogen-induced disconnection of the circuit responsible for cyclic drive of gonadotrophin secretion.

Progesterone interactions

Little research has been done concerning the interactions of progesterone with the brain. The results reported do not indicate a specific progesterone interaction in the rat.

Knowledge of the effects of prenatal and early postnatal hormone exposure of the human, is restricted to observations in subjects exposed to abnormally high or low levels of sex hormones. These can occur because of endocrine abnormalities of the foetus, hormone-producing tumours in the mother, and hormone treatment during pregnancy (Ehrhardt 1978; Meyer Bahlburg 1978). Some of such experiences are used to support much disputed claims that exposure in the first trimester of pregnancy to natural hormones or synthetic equivalents, can have long-term effects on the intelligence quotient (IQ), on educational attainments (Dalton 1976; Meyer Bahlburg 1978), and on personality, and/or temperament (Reinisch and Karow 1977). Other experiments, together with evidence from animal studies, emphasize the possible dangers of hormone treatment in pregnancy. Administered during critical stages of development, sex hormones can play a major role in determining the rate of maturation and differentiation of the CNS.

BIOCHEMICAL EFFECTS

The mechanism of action of sex steroids in the brain at the molecular level is unknown.

Respiration and metabolism of brain tissue

Steroidal control of cerebral metabolism has been demonstrated in rats and in man (Gordan 1956; Gordan, Bentinck, and Eisenberg 1951). Large doses of progestins have a powerful anaesthetizing action. Some progestational compounds produce in man a profound reduction in cerebral blood flow, in oxygen, and in glucose consumption, comparable to that found in barbiturate anaesthesia. Parallels between the anaesthetic action of steroids and their ability to inhibit glucose oxidation of rat brain homogenates have been found for progesterone and α-oestradiol, but not for stilboestrol. This non-steroidal oestrogen is less anaesthetic but the most potent brain respiration inhibitor; it may exert its effect by competing with cytocrome c as a hydrogen acceptor for lactic dihydrogenase.

Testosterone inhibits the oxygen uptake of rat brain and exerts a 'braking' action upon the oxidation of glucose by rat brain (Eisenberg, Gordan, and Elliott (1949). The elevated cerebral oxygen and glucose consumption found in castrated pre-pubertal rats and in pre-adolescent eunuchoidism, is restored to approximately normal by administration, *in vivo*, of progesterone or androgens, but not by 17-β-oestradiol. The steep fall in cerebral metabolic rate at puberty is possibly the result of the increased production of steroid hormones such as androgens and corticosteroids.

Water and electrolytes

Perhaps one of the primary important effects of all hormones, including the sex hormones, is directly concerned with the regulation of water and electrolyte metabolism. Most hormones affect calcium metabolism directly or indirectly, and because of this, are thought to exert important effects on brain maturation, behaviour, and excitability; although the latter can also be influenced via other mechanisms. Effects on calcium metabolism have been demonstrated for oestrogens in a variety of species.

Protein metabolism

Hormones can influence protein metabolism of nervous tissues, via enzymes directly involved in protein synthesis, via indirect effects on RNA metabolism, by affecting transport/metabolism of amino acids, or by an influence on the cell. They increase RNA synthesis, or synthesis of selective RNAs at least, in peripheral organs concerned with reproduction. Hormones may also affect the transport or metabolism of amino acids or influence the energy metabolism of the cell. Oestrogens have been found to increase protein synthesis in the cerebral cortex of oophorectomized guinea pigs. Whether progestins and androgenic-anabolic steroids influence the protein metabolism of the brain still has to be established.

Enzymes and neurotransmitters

Oestrogens reduce, in a dose-dependent manner, monoamine oxidase (MAO) activity in various brain regions, in plasma and in platelets. Choline acetylase, on the other hand, is influenced by oestrogens in the reverse manner. Various other enzymes, including catechol-*o*-methyltransferase, glucose 6-phosphate dihydrogenase, isocitrate dihydrogenase, and malate dihydrogenase are also affected by oestrogens, as is the secretion and re-uptake of neurotransmitters such as noradrenaline, serotonin, and dopamine, and their receptors are also affected by oestrogens. As a consequence they all vary during the cycle, in pregnancy, after gonadectomy, and perhaps also after hypophysectomy. These effects, particularly on brain amines, might be mediated by gonadotrophins, but direct effects on turnover, increased amine synthesis and decreased uptake of noradrenaline and 5-HT, have also been reported for oestrogens and the aromatizable testosterone.

Since sex hormones affect amine metabolism and behaviour, the two may be linked, although the question as to whether there is indeed a causal relationship between these alterations in brain amines and sexual behaviour, remains to be answered. In male and female mammals depression of 5-HT activity in the CNS induces sexual behaviour. Elevation of dopamine levels in males and depression thereof in females, act in a similar manner. A possible beneficial effect of oestrogens on tardative and L-DOPA-induced dyskinesias, was thought to be related to their assumed antidopaminergic activity. Hormone dependent changes were also observed in tryptophan and γ-aminobutyric acid (GABA) metabolism, although it appears that changes of adrenaline or noradrenaline have little effect on behaviour.

Progesterone is reported to reduce 5-HT uptake, increase 5-HT turnover, lower the brain aminobutyric acid (GABA) content, and to counteract its increase after oophorectomy. Others suggest that progesterone activates a noradrenergic system in the hypothalamus, by causing release of noradrenaline or by sensitizing noradrenaline receptors in postsynaptic membranes. Some data indicate that progesterone may activate dopaminergic systems; thus inhibition of lordosis could be due to a dopamine-induced increase in locomotor activity (Feder and Marrone 1977).

Testosterone increases the septal concentration of GABA in castrated rats and by this is thought to diminish the inconsistency, distractibility, and greater variability in day-to-day performance (Earley and Leonard 1979). Testosterone affects brain monoamine metabolism and may also be responsible for some changes in brain 5-HT concentration which accompany sexual maturity (Kendall and Tonge 1976). The influence of endogenous and exogenous testosterone on the hypothalamic modulation of LH synthesis and/or liberation, is a further indication for its action on the CNS.

EFFECTS ON BRAIN FUNCTIONS

Regulation of ovulation

High sensitivity to the negative feed-back actions of sex steroids probably controls prepubertal gonadotrophin secretion. In the rat, a sudden change in the hypothalamic threshold to the gonadotrophin-inhibiting effect of oestrogens, over a narrow range of time near the onset of puberty, has been observed. This decline in sensitivity is the principal factor that initiates puberty.

Sex hormones modulate hypothalamic-releasing factors and pituitary gonadotrophins, by direct action on the pituitary and by feed-back mechanisms. The elevated midcyclic plasma oestrogen level provokes, presumably via discharge of LHRF and synchronized with an increased pituitary sensitivity to LHRF, the preovulatory surge of LH and FSH secretion which is most probably responsible for ovulation.

Posture and locomotion

In castrated adult female rats, oestrogens promote a typical respective behaviour pattern; when mounted by a male they assume a lordotic position. This effect on sexual receptivity can also be produced in castrated males, be it only with much higher doses. Predominantly, areas in the anterior hypothalamus and the preoptic region are held responsible for this oestrogen-induced lordosis, and involvement of changes of MAO activity might be of relevance. Progesterone can either facilitate or reduce this oestrogen effect, depending on the sequence of administration of the hormones. Oestrogens may activate both excitatory and inhibitory neural substrates for locomotion. There seems to be a fundamental relationship between lordosis and locomotion and between these two phenomena and the limbic–hypothalamic system.

The decreased tonus and electromyographic activity of abdominal muscles during pregnancy or following treatment with progestins might be caused by a central action of these steroids. This action is thought to favour development of compensatory lordosis in pregnancy.

The senses and food intake

Gonadal steriods might have an effect on thresholds for taste, smell, and hearing, but many more studies are required to substantiate this. Food intake shows cyclic variations and, in particular, artificial oestrogens have been found to reduce food intake (Spiteri, Drewett, and Padel 1980).

Body temperature and respiration

A close relationship between the temperature regulating mechanisms and the endocrine system is very likely. There is a rise in body temperature in women at the time of ovulation, persisting until menstruation, and in pregnancy the body temperature remains elevated during the first half of gestation. This thermogenetic action is also seen after administration of natural or artificial progestins in non-ovulating women and in men. It is most probably caused by a direct or indirect effect on a thermogenetic centre in the hypothalamus. The 5-β-OH steroid hormone metabolites etiocholanolon, pregnenolone, and 11ketopregnanolone, also cause a rise of body temperature in humans, though a frank fever producing action of these steroid metabolites seems to be highly species-specific.

The carbon dioxide sensitivity of the respiratory centre increases in the normal cycle after ovulation and in the second half of pregnancy. Respiratory stimulation can likewise be produced by administration of progestins to both women and men. Similar effects have also been observed with oestrogens.

The biological clock

Various recurring rhythmic biological and behavioural events, such as ovulation and menstrual cycles, are regulated by mechanisms more primitive than homeostasis. These suggested 'biological clock mechanisms' are hardly affected by internal and external influences, with the exception of light. Endocrinological changes such as gonadectomy, mating, pregnancy, lactation, or hypophysectomy, have been reported to be without effect on the 'biological clock'.

ELECTROPHYSIOLOGICAL EFFECTS

Brain excitability

Brain excitability is markedly and differentially influenced by sex hormones, oestrogens having an excitatory effect. The electroshock threshold (EST) is lower in female rats than in males, and it fluctuates with the phases of the menstrual cycle, reaching the lowest level at ovulation. A decrease in EST can be produced in a dose-dependent fashion by oestrogen administration. This effect is assumed to be mediated by mechanisms other than electrolyte changes, since EST has been found to be lowered by oestrogen, in spite of elevated plasma sodium concentrations and increased extracellular/intracellular sodium ratio in the cerebral cortex. The micro-electroshock seizure threshold in different parts of the brain reacts differently to oestrogens, increasing in some parts, decreasing in others.

Various steroid hormones including progesterone and in a much less pronounced fashion, androgens, have an anaesthetic effect in a number of animals; in large doses they produce deep anaesthesia (Gordan, Guadagni, Picchi, and Adams 1956; Selye 1941). Steroids inhibit the rate of oxygen and glucose uptake by the brain; this inhibition is held to be a physiological phenomenon and can be used for surgical anaesthesia (Gordan 1956). In man, progesterone has a soporific effect. It has been shown that the CNS depressant effect of progesterone surpasses that of short acting barbiturates, and the related 5β-pregnane derivatives are even more potent in depressing arousal from reticular formation stimulation, than hydroxydione and pentobarbital (Gyermek, Genther, and Fleming 1967). The hemisuccinate ester of the steroid 21-hydroxy-pregnane-dione-3,20, given intravenously to human subjects, produces anaesthesia and cerebral metabolic changes identical with those produced by barbiturates, but without respiratory depression (Gordan *et al*. 1956). The anaesthetic activity of these steroids can be dissociated from their hormonal activity by structural modification of the molecule.

An increased epileptogenic activity has been observed after injection or cortical application of an oestrogen. Progesterone raises the EST. The threshold of cortical EEG arousal on direct stimulation of the hypothalamus is much increased by progesterone, while the elevation of the threshold on stimulation of the reticular formation is not as large. In patients with partial epilepsy, a very low number of generalized seizures has been recorded during periods of high progesterone levels, whereas many seizures occurred during the follicular phase, and after rapid decrease of the progesterone level following menstruation. This is in accordance with the beneficial effect of progesterone on seizures that has been so repeatedly supposed, and the claimed epileptogenic effect of oestrogens in epileptics. Progesterone seems to be an anticonvulsive agent.

Electrical activity and sleep

A number of pre- and post-ovulatory differences in the EEG observed in animals and in man may be linked with effects of sex hormones. However, the reported observations are far from uniform. Under oestrogen treatment, driving response rates to photic stimulation were inhibited in amenorrhoeic and in depressed women. A similar suppression of EEG driving, i.e. facilitation of EEG resistance to photic stimulation (inhibition of the tendency of EEG rhythm to be evoked by a flashing light), was found with androgens (Stenn, Klaiber, Vogel, and Broverman 1972). This reaction is similar to that observed after treatment with adrenergic substances, and a possible relationship with suppression of increased MAO activity is suggested. Some studies indicate that androgens can facilitate sexual reflexes, others that they have a protective effect against increased brain excitability.

Power spectral analysis of the EEG shows that the α-rhythm is slightly but significantly accelerated in the luteal phase, with a maximum shortly before menstruation (Itil *et al.* 1976). Some investigators have observed changes in the ratio between theta waves and total activity of the frontal lobes during the menstrual cycle, with the lowest ratio during the luteal phase. It has also been reported that sufficient slowing of the EEG occurs in association with menstruation to convert a normal EEG to an abnormal one. In the final weeks of pregnancy when progesterone levels are high, the EEG is low compared to post-partum tracings. However, the postmenopausal EEG is not significantly altered by progestins or stilboestrol. Oestrogen effects in the quantitative pharmaco-electroencephalogram (CEEG) are similar to those of tricyclic antidepressants, whereas progestagens cause changes of the profile resembling those of minor tranquillizers (Herrman and Beach 1978*a,b*).

In guinea pigs, hormone induced oestrus is accompanied by a decrease in the amounts of both paradoxical (REM) and slow wave sleep; in rabbits oestrogens increase total sleeping time and REM sleep; while in the intact cat, large doses of oestrogens produce no significant change in cortical electrical activity. Perimenopausal women treated with an oestrogen showed more REM sleep and significantly reduced intervening wakefulness.

Effects on single neurones

In the lateral anterior hypothalamic areas, oestrogens enhance the inhibitory responsiveness to pain, cold, and cervical stimuli, whereas in the septum they decrease the number of inhibitory responses. Exogenous or endogenous progesterone selectively depresses the excitation of hypothalamic neurones by stimuli from the genital tract; this effect might be related to the effect of progesterone on 5-HT metabolism (Ladisich 1977).

EFFECTS ON BEHAVIOUR

Human behaviour is a result of interactions between physiological, psychological, and social parameters. In consequence, and also because of lack of relevant scientifically valid experimental data, it is not surprising that the highly complex relationship between hormones and behaviour is still a matter of intense controversy. The part played by sex hormones in the direct control of overt human behaviour is, compared with that found in lower animals, slight, and less readily definable, though one generally assumes that hormones affect behaviour through actions mediated by the CNS. In man these hormones though necessary for maintenance of libido and sexual behaviour, seem to control the intensity of such behaviour rather than its direction. Their most pronounced influence on behaviour is perhaps on psychological (emotional rather than intellectual) and sociological aspects (Eayrs and Glass 1962). In foetal or neonatal life, sex hormones organize the sexually undifferentiated brain, with regard to neuroendocrine function and patterns of not only sexual but also non-sexual behaviour.

In castrated male rats, oestrogens inhibit the production of sexual excitement by androgens, and cause the animals to exhibit female sexual behaviour (lordosis). In sufficiently high doses, oestradiol activates the complete male copulatory pattern including ejaculation. Oestrogens, like aromatizable androgens, augment mating behaviour in oophorectomized rhesus monkeys by increasing proceptivity, but are without effect on receptivity. With a constant dose of progesterone, the stimulating effects on both proceptive and receptive behaviour have been found to be oestrogen dose-dependent in ovariectomized Syrian hamsters (Steel 1981) and rats (Spiteri *et al*. 1980). Others have reported proceptivity increasing with progesterone in a dose-dependent fashion (Tennent, Smith, and Davidson 1980).

Oestrogens stimulate aggressiveness, not only in relation to mating behaviour but also towards a third individual and inanimate objects. Additional progesterone decreases aggressiveness in relation to mating behaviour, and in particular the aggressiveness towards a third individual. Oestrogens decrease fearfulness, influence conditioned taste aversion, delay extinction, and counteract some behavioural effects of *d*-amphetamine in rodents.

Mood and menses

There are significant fluctuations in mood, mental content, and outlook during the menstrual cycle. These are thought to be related to concomitant hormonal changes, but the available research data are insufficient to characterize beyond doubt the effects of physiological concentrations of female sex hormones on psychic function in woman (Kopera 1973). It is assumed that oestrogens account at least in part for the increased well-being, alertness, and vigour that occur in the first half of the menstrual cycle. At the same time, an active extrovert heterosexual drive, with an ovulatory peak in sexual attractiveness and both female-initiated autosexual and heterosexual activity, has been demonstrated (Adams, Gold, and Burt 1978). However, there is no convincing evidence that administration of oestrogens would appreciably increase sexual drive in the normal woman. This is consistent with the observation that neither physiological ovarian failure at menopause nor ovariectomy alters sexual behaviour dramatically; this is only the case when all sources of endogenous androgens and oestrogens are removed by adrenalectomy. That constrasts drastically with the situation in subprimate females, where ovariectomy is mostly followed by a complete loss in mating behaviour.

Exposure in childhood

Recent studies indicate that children prenatally exposed to more oestrogens than progestins exhibit effects on the personality in that they are more group-oriented and group-dependent, less individualistic, and less self-sufficient; they are more 'outer' or 'other' directed (Reinisch and Karow 1977). Some fall behind in psychological maturation, and experience anxiety and serious behaviour problems (Ehrhardt 1978; Reinisch and Karow 1977). There seems to be a physiological predisposition towards hyperoestrogenism in puberty, and in some individuals prolonged mental stress can produce hyperoestrogenism. In these subjects deterioration in school achievement, social hyperactivity, hypochondria, inhibited aggression, sexual problems, increased sensitivity, and exhaustion following prolonged intrapsychic conflict have been reported.

In rats ovariectomized at birth, early treatment with physiological amounts of oestrogens produces feminine open-field behaviour; however, administration of unphysiologically high doses produces paradoxically masculinizing effects. This suggests that high doses of oestrogens can reach the subcortical brain regions concerned with motivation, emotion, and sexual behaviour, where its action is masculinizing. An excess of oestrogens in genetic males is said to be associated with reduced athletic skill, lowered aggressiveness and assertiveness, and retarded heterosexual development (Meyer Bahlburg 1978).

Oestrogens in adults

In men treated with high doses of oestrogens as indicated for diseases such as prostatic carcinoma, loss of sexual desire and potency, longing for asexual tenderness, mood changes towards depression, reduced drive, and inactivity are observed. Only occasionally hyperactivity and euphoria to explosiveness are recorded. Trials to improve mental functioning in conditions such as cerebral thrombosis or atherosclerosis, using higher doses of oestrogens, have not demonstrated pronounced beneficial effects. Recently high doses of oestrogens have been claimed to exert an antidepressant effect comparable to that of tricyclic antidepressants (Herrmann and Beach 1978a). Whether they are indeed therapeutically useful to relieve chronic severe, intransigent states of depression, by influences upon central adrenergic functioning, still has to be confirmed.

Oestrogen deficiency as found in women with inadequately developed sexual organs, as for example in Turner's syndrome, causes psychosexual infantility. The psychological characteristics of these patients are described as being warm and friendly, they are naive, lack aggression, and obtain little satisfaction from sexual activity. These symptoms respond to oestrogen administration.

In castrated women, the psychological changes caused by the oestrogen deficiency are usually more regular, but of shorter duration and less severe than those in climacteric woman, in whom oestrogen production diminishes gradually. In neither instance is it possible to observe a sudden reduction or abolition of erotic imagery, sensations, or active sexual behaviour (drive and response), though a variety of psychic disturbances accompany the postmenopausal years. Obviously, many of these psychic alterations are unconnected with the progressive oestrogen deficiency. However, in some the hormonal imbalance seems to be of importance. This can be deduced from a number of recent investigations in which reproducible psychometric methods were employed. The observations clearly indicate a beneficial prophylactic and therapeutic effect of oestrogens on some psychic functions. Improvements have been seen in psychomotor coordination, in concentration, attention, information processing capacity, irritability, anxiety, and in some parameters of alertness.

Few reports suggest that oestrogens improve social behaviour or prevent expected deterioration of mental performance, as evidenced by some perceptual, attentional, and memory processes, although others dispute such effects. Some investigations suggest that oestrogens display effects usually associated with psychostimulants (Herrmann and Beach 1978a). Above all, however, the most beneficial and frequently observed therapeutic action of oestrogens in a mood-elevating, psychotonic effect, which often causes a sense of exceptional well-being and vigour, most probably due to restoration of somatic efficiency and psychic equilibrium.

Progesterone in adults

In a wide variety of non-primates, oestrogens activate female behaviour. A similar effect of progesterone varies markedly among species, can be absent altogether, and in some non-primates progesterone suppresses female sexual behaviour. Thus animal experiments indicate that progesterone can have either facilitatory or inhibitory influences on female sexual behaviour (Feder and Marrone 1977). It may interact with oestrogens in facilitating sexual responses in different temporal sequences in different species but can also cause inhibition of sexual behaviour. The latter effect depends on whether the oestrogen conditioning is complete and accompanied by a low level of progesterone (sequential); or whether oestrogen conditioning is incomplete and accompanied by a high level of progesterone (concurrent). Oestrogens promote female's sexual attractiveness whilst progesterone makes females sexually less attractive. Progestins can delay extinction of conditioned avoidance in the rat, and cats under long-term administration of a progestagen are more docile and easier to trap.

There is some indication that noradrenergic mechanisms are involved in the facilitation of sexual behaviour by progesterone, but other neurotransmitters are likely to be also of importance. The inhibitory effects of progestins on oestrogen-dependent processes, are thought to be indirect. They appear to depend more on transference of information from progesterone-responsive cells to oestrogen-responsive cells, than on direct impedance of intranuclear programming processes in oestrogen-sensitive cells (Feder and Marrone 1977).

The available evidence concerning the psychological changes thought to be associated with progestins in man is very incomplete and conflicting. Based on observations during the menstrual cycle, in pregnancy, and on administration of progestational substances, one concludes that these compounds would cause low libido, tiredness, reduced activity; would lower the incidence of emotional instability, impulsiveness, and irritability; might be involved in premenstrual tension, and would provoke tension, anxiety, depression, and occasionally even psychotic episodes. However, this common belief has been questioned by opposing findings. Some psychopharmacological studies in the luteal phase or with progestins, indicate an increase in reaction time, performance speed and quality and an anti-anxiety effect. There is also favourable influence on instinctive maternal tendencies, as expressed in dreams, such as higher obvious and symbolic maternal scores.

Progestagens used as anti-androgens in the treatment of sex offenders, have a mood-stabilizing, mildly sedative effect. Progestagens block the impairment of performance caused by LSD, via a mechanism which is not yet elucidated. Studies with the computerized electro-encephalogram (CEEG), suggest that some progestins have a profile similar to that of a minor tranquillizer. This is consistent with the observation that progestins have sedative-tranquillizing properties, and in high i.v. doses an anaesthesia-like effect. It is also in agreement with the assumption that progesterone has a protective effect against stress reactions (Ladisich 1977), and is compatible with the repeated observation that progestagens can diminish aggressive behaviour and can have a mood-equilibrating effect. Such properties are occasionally used in the treatment of psychiatric patients (Lydeken 1979).

The claim that prenatal administration of progesterone enhances intelligence and improves educational attainments (Dalton 1975, 1976), meets much criticism and is still a matter of debate (Sachar 1976). It seems, however, that prenatal exposure to mainly progestagens affects personality; children of mothers given progestagens for the maintenance of at-risk pregnancies, were found to be significantly more independent, sensitive, individualistic, self-assured and self-sufficient. Furthermore, they were more 'inner' or 'self' directed, they showed less aggressiveness and athletic skills, and a significant preference for attractive stylish clothes (Ehrhardt 1978; Reinisch and Karow 1977). Sons of diabetic mothers who were treated with oestrogens and progestagens during pregnancy were less masculine, aggressive-assertive, and athletically able than controls (Yalom, Green, and Fisk 1973).

Effects of androgens

Pre- and perinatal androgens have a profound effect on sexual and non-sexual behaviour patterns in rodents and primates. A prenatal excess of male hormones in genetic females has been reported to be associated with tomboyish behaviour. This is evidenced by a high level of energy expenditure in play, an increased interest in athletics, a reduced interest in dolls and clothes, a low level of maternalism, and an increased interest in an adult career as contrasted with marriage and motherhood. It is undecided whether this is the result of an androgenic effect on the brain, or whether it is related to postnatal factors (Quadagno and Briscoe 1977). Perinatal androgen excess in man does not confer a postnatal IQ advantage as has been speculated previously.

In some situations androgens potentiate aggressive behaviour in animals (there are much less data from the human), but there is a considerable individual dissociation between androgen levels and sexual or aggressive behaviour. Hence such effects of androgens must certainly not be expected under all circumstances. This makes it necessary to refer to the effects of androgens on sexual or aggressive behaviour only together with elaboration of social factors, and the behaviour pattern and its antecedent conditions (Connor 1972; Rose 1980). Aggressive behaviour in ovariectomized hamsters is only induced by aromatizable androgens such as testosterone, but not by dihydrotestosterone. This suggests that the androgen is aromatized before acting on the CNS (Rudolph 1976). Testosterone is assumed to have a permissive influence, in that it increases the propensity to behave sexually or aggressively. However, other factors, particularly social ones, seem to determine the final expression of any sexual or aggressive behaviour (Rose 1980).

In the human, administration of an androgen has been found to enhance activity and performance of automized cognitive tests, and in ageing males decreases neuroticism whilst increasing extroversion as well as masculine self-image (Kaiser, Kies, Maass, Schmidt, Beach, Bormacher, Herrmann, and Richter 1978). Androgens appear to affect brain function, as evidenced by the EEG and by cognition status, in a manner similar to a mild central adrenergic stimulant. Whether this adrenergic effect is achieved via inhibition of monoamine oxidase is still under discussion.

Although androgens are not the exclusive basis of libidinous urge, which is multidetermined, they are claimed to be the hormones of eroticism, mainly determining sexual appetite in men and women. Erotic imagery, sensations, and actions are most probably maintained in a state of satisfactory functioning in men and women by androgens. Perhaps they influence libido by affecting end-organ sensitivity (Young and Corner 1961). Excess of androgens in women causes increased libido.

Castration

Castration of male animals does not lead to immediate cessation of copulation and in higher mammals it does not markedly impair behaviour for some time. Obviously, androgens and experience are necessary for the full expression of sex behaviour. In man, androgens play a major role in initiating and maintaining sexual function. There is little systematic information on the rate of decline, or the physiological factors affecting the loss of behavioural responses with age (Davidson 1972). However, castration of the adult man is followed by a decline in libido and sexual activity, either fairly rapidly or in the course of years. Castration does not lead to a fall in aggressiveness (Rose 1977). Castration before puberty results in lack of development of sexual behaviour. These effects can be prevented by androgens. It appears that sexual potency in men can only be improved by androgen therapy in cases of androgen deficiency (Bancroft and Wu 1982; Skakkebaek, Bancroft, Davidson; Warner 1981; Wu, Bancroft, Davidson, and Nicol 1982), but either not at all or to hardly any extent, when androgen levels are normal (Benkert, Witt, Adam, and Leitz 1979).

Psychic effects

The evidence reported so far on the psychic effects of sex hormones is certainly insufficient to enable any final conclusions to be made. This also holds true for the numerous and conflicting observations in women using contraceptive preparations, which contain a progestin or the combination of an oestrogen with a progestagen, as active compounds. In this field the methodological difficulties are formidable, hence a large literature with contradictory viewpoints exists on the subject. Nevertheless, the majority of data strongly support the conventional idea that oestrogens are somewhat stimulant, induce activity, cause irritability, and worsen premenstrual tension; while the progestins seem to cause passivity, mood changes towards depression, and relieve premenstrual irritability. However, the great diversity of partly unidentifiable factors contributing to the net result of psychic influences of sex hormones, prevents the isolation of specific effects of any single hormonal substance.

CONCLUSIONS

Results of animal experiments and experiences in man indicate that the brain is certainly one of the target organs of sex hormones. Hormone uptake, distribution, and binding is differential in various areas of the CNS. Specific receptors for oestrogens and progestins, but not (yet) for androgens, have been identified in the brain. The mechanism of action at the molecular level is still obscure. However, an appreciable number of data concerning effects on respiration and metabolism of brain tissue, on water and electrolyte balance, protein metabolism, enzyme activities, and on neurotransmitters, are available.

The influence of gonadal hormones on the brain in pre- and perinatal periods, is responsible for sexual differentiation and endocrine functions of the CNS. In postnatal life sex steroids regulate ovulation, affect posture, locomotion, temperature regulation, and respiration; they interfere with the excitability and electrical activity of the brain and with sleep. Undoubtedly, gonadal hormones and their artificial equivalents exert profound influences on brain functions. With our present knowledge, it seems rather hazardous, however, to predict the therapeutic applicability of these effects for pathological conditions, with the exception of their use to supplement deficiencies.

References

Adams, D. B., Gold, A. R., and Burt, A. D. (1978). Rise in female-initiated sexual activity at ovulation and its suppression by oral contraceptives. *N. Engl. J. Med.* **299**, 1145–50.

Arai, Y. (1981). Synaptic correlates of sexual differentiation. *Trends Neurosci.* **4**, 291–3.

Arnold, A. B. (1980). Sexual differences in the brain. *Am. Sci.* **68**, 165–73.

Bäckström, T. (1977). Estrogen and progesterone in relation to different activities in the central nervous system. *Acta Obstet. Gynecol. Scand.* **66** (Suppl.), 1–17.

Bancroft, J. and Wu, F. C. (1982). Changes in erectile responsiveness during androgen replacement therapy. *Arch. Sex. Behav.* **12**, 59–66.

Benkert, O., Witt, W., Adam, W., and Leitz, A. (1979). Effects of testosterone undecanoate on sexual potency and the hypothalamic-pituitary-gonadal axis of impotent males. *Arch. Sex. Behav.* **8**, 471–9.

Booth, J. E. (1978). Effects of the aromatization inhibitor androst-4-ene-3,6,17-trione on sexual differentiation induced by testosterone in the neonatally castrated rat. *J. Endocrinol.* **79**, 69–76.

Connor, R. L. (1972). Hormones, biogenic amines and aggression. In *Hormones and behavior* (ed. S. Levine) pp. 209–33. Academic Press, New York.

Dalton, K. (1975). The effect of progesterone on brain function. *Acta Endocrinol.* (Suppl.) **199**, 49–50.

—— (1976). Prenatal progesterone and educational attainments. *Br. J. Psychiatr.* **129**, 438–42.

Davidson, J. M. (1972). Hormones and reproductive behavior. In *Hormones and behavior* (ed. S. Levine) pp. 63–103. Academic Press, New York.

Dörner, G. (1979). Hormones, brain differentiation and sexuality. In *Emotion and reproduction*, Pt. A, *Proceedings of a Congress, Rome 1977*, (ed. L. Carenza and L. Zichella) pp. 519–528. Academic Press, London.

Earley, C. J. and Leonard, B. E. (1979). The effects of castration and hormone replacement on runway behavior and GABA concentrations in the septum. *Irish J. Med. Sci.* 148, 227–31.

Eayrs, J. T. and Glass, A. (1962). The ovary and behaviour. In *The ovary* (eds. S. Zuckerman, A. M. Mandl, P. Eckstein) pp. 381–433. Academic Press, New York.

Editorial (1979). Sexual behaviour and the sex hormones. *Lancet* 2, 17–18.

Ehrhardt, A. A. (1978). Behavioral effects of estrogen in the human female. *Pediatrics* 62, 1166–70.

Eisenberg, E., Gordan, G. S., and Elliott, H. W. (1949). The effect of castration and of testosterone upon the respiration of rat brain. *Science* 109, 337–8.

Eisenfeld, A. J. (1972). Interaction of estrogens, progestational agents, and androgens with brain and pituitary and their role in the control of ovulation. In *Perspectives in neuropharmacology* (ed. S. H. Snyder) pp. 113–42. Oxford University Press, New York.

Feder, H. H. and Marrone, B. L. (1977). Progesterone: its role in the central nervous system as a facilitator and inhibitor of sexual behavior and gonadotrophin release. *Ann. N.Y. Acad. Sci.* 206, 331–54.

Fishman, J. (1977). The catechol estrogens. *Neuroendocrinology* 22, 363–74.

Gordan, G. S. (1956). II. Hormones and metabolism. Influence of steroids on cerebral metabolism in man. *Recent Progr. Hormone Res.* 12, 153–74.

—— Bentinck, R. C., and Eisenberg, E. (1951). The influence of steroids on cerebral metabolism. *Ann. N.Y. Acad. Sci.* 54, 575–607.

—— Guadagni, N., Picchi, J., and Adams, J. E. (1956). Steroid anaesthesia in man: clinical and cerebral metabolic effects. *J. Int. Coll. Surg.* 25, 9–12.

Goy, R. W. and McEwen, B. S. (1980). *Sexual differentiation of the brain*. MIT Press, Cambridge, MA.

Gyermek, L., Genther, G., and Fleming, N. (1967). Some effects of progesterone and related steroids on the central nervous system. *Int. J. Neuropharmac.* 6, 191–8.

Herbert, J. (1977). Hormones and sexual behaviour in adulthood. In *Handbook of sexology* (eds. J. Money and H. Musaph), pp. 375–492. Excerpta Medica, Amsterdam.

Herrmann, W. M. and Beach, R. C. (1978a). The psychotropic properties of estrogens. *Pharmakopsychiat.* 11, 164–76.

—— —— (1978b). Experimental and clinical data indicating the psychotropic properties of progestogens. *Postgrad. Med. J.* 54 (Suppl. 2), 82–7.

Itil, T. M., Laudahn, G., and Herrmann, W. M. (eds., 1976). *Psychotropic action of hormones*. Spectrum, New York.

Junkmann, K. (ed.) (1968/69). *Handbuch der experimentellen Pharmakologie. Die Gestagene*. Vol. XII/1 (1968), Vol. XII/2 (1969). Springer, Berlin.

Kaiser, E., Kies, N., Maass, G., Schmidt, H., Beach, R. C., Bormacher, K., Herrmann, W. M., and Richter, E. (1978). The measurement of the psychotropic effects of an androgen in aging males with psychovegetative symptomatology: a controlled double blind study mesterolone versus placebo. *Prog. Neuro-Psychopharmac.* 2, 505–15.

Kendall, D. and Tonge, S. (1976). Monoamine concentrations in eight areas of the brain of mature and immature male rats and effects of injected hormones. *J. Pharm. Pharmac.* 28, Suppl., 37P.

Kopera, H. (1973). Estrogens and psychic function. In *Ageing and estrogens. Frontiers of Hormone Research*, vol. 2, pp. 118–33. Karger, Basel.

—— (1980). Female hormones and brain function. In *Hormones and the brain* (eds. D. de Wied and P. A. van Keep) pp. 189–203. MTP Press, Lancaster.

Ladisich, W. (1977). Influence of progesterone on serotonin metabolism: a possible causal factor for mood changes. *Psychoneuroendocrinology* 2, 257–66.

Lisk, R. D. and Reuter, L. A. (1977). *In vivo* progesterone treatment enhances (^{3}H) estradiol retention by neural tissue of the female rat. *Endocrinology* 100, 1652–58.

Lydeken, K. (1979). Experiences with the use of long-term Lynestrenol in the treatment of mentally handicapped patients. *Br. J. Fam. Plan.* 14 (4), 15–16.

MacLusky, N. J. and McEwen, B. S. (1978). Oestrogen modulates progestin receptor concentrations in some rat brain regions but not in others. *Nature, Lond.* 274, 276–8.

McDonald, P., Tan, H. S., Beyer, C., Sampson, C., Newton, F., Kitching, P., Bresci, B., Greenhill, R., Baker, R., and Pritchard, D. (1970). Failure of 5α-dihydrotestosterone to initiate sexual behaviour in the castrated male rat. *Nature, Lond.* 227, 964–5.

McEwen, B. S. and Parsons, B. (1982). Gonadal steroid action on the brain: neurochemistry and neuropharmacology. *Ann. Rev. Pharmac. Toxicol.* 22, 555–98.

Meyer Bahlburg, H. F. L. (1978). Behavioral effects of estrogen treatment in human males. *Pediatrics* 62, 1171–7.

Naftolin, F., Ryan, K. J., Davies, I. J., Reddy, V. V., Flores, F., Petro, Z., and Kuhn, M. (1975). The formation of estrogens by central neuroendocrine tissues. In *Recent progress in hormone research* (ed. R. O. Greep), Vol. 31. pp. 295–319. Academic Press, New York.

Paul, S. M. and Axelrod, J. (1977). Catechol estrogens: Presence in brain and endocrine tissues. *Science* 197, 657–9.

Porter, R. and Whelan, J. (eds.) (1979). *Sex, hormones and behaviour*. Ciba Foundation Symposium 62 (new series). Excerpta Medica, Amsterdam.

Quadagno, D. M. and Briscoe, R. (1977). Effect of perinatal gonadal hormones on selected nonsexual behavior patterns: a critical assessment of the non-human and human literature. *Psychol. Bull.* 84, 62–80.

Reinisch, J. M. and Karow, W. G. (1977). Prenatal exposure to synthetic progestins and estrogens: effects on human development. *Arch. Sex. Behav.* 6, 257–88.

Rose, R. M. (1977). Neuroendocrine correlates of sexual and aggressive behaviour in humans. In *Psychopharmacology: a generation of progress* (eds. M. A. Lipton, A. DiMascio, and K. F. Killam). Raven Press, New York.

—— (1980). Androgens and behaviour. In *Hormones and the brain* (eds. D. de Wied and P. A. van Keep) pp. 175–87. MTP Press, Lancaster.

Rudolph, B. A. (1976). The effect of testosterone, dihydrotestosterone, estrogen and nitromifene citrate on aggressive behaviour in female hamsters. *Dissertation Abstr. Intern.* B 36, No. 12, Pt. 1, 6434.

Sachar, E. J. (ed.) (1976). *Hormones, behavior and psychopathology*. Raven Press, New York.

Sawyer, C. H. and Gorski, R. A. (eds.) (1971). *Steroid hormones and brain function*. University of California Press, Berkeley, CA.

Selye, H. (1941). Anesthetic effect of steroid hormones. *Proc. Soc. Exp. Biol. Med.* 46, 116.

Skakkebaek, B., Bancroft, J., Davidson, D. W., and Warner, P. (1981). Androgen replacement with oral testosterone undecanoate in hypogonadal men: a double blind controlled study. *Clin. Endocrinol.* 14, 49–61.

Spiteri, N. J., Drewett, R. F., and Padel, U. (1980). Behavioral effects of ethynyl estrogens in the female rat. *Physiol. Behav.* 25, 409-15.

Steel, E. (1981). Control of proceptive and receptive behavior by ovarian hormones in the Syrian hamster (Mesocricetus auratus). *Hormones Behav.* 15, 141-56.

Stenn, P. G., Klaiber, E. L., Vogel, W., and Broverman, D. M. (1972). Testosterone effects upon photic stimulation of the electroencephalogram (EEG) and mental performance of humans. *Percept. Motor Skills* 34, 371-8.

Stumpf, W. E., Sar, M., and Keefer, D. A. (1975). Anatomical distribution of estrogen in the central nervous system of mouse, rat, tree shrew, and squirrel monkey. In *Advances in the biosciences* (ed. G. Raspé) pp. 77-86. Pergamon Press, Oxford.

Tausk, M. and de Visser, J. (1971). Various other effects of progesterone. In *International encyclopaedia of pharmacology* (ed. M. Tausk) vol. 48, pp. 375-87. Pergamon Press, Oxford.

Tennent, B. J., Smith, E. R., and Davidson, J. M. (1980). The effects of estrogen and progesterone on female rat proceptive behavior. *Hormones Behav.* 14, 65-75.

Vernikos-Danellis, J. (1972). Effects of hormones on the central nervous system. In *Hormones and behaviour* (ed. S. Levine) pp. 11-62. Academic Press, New York.

Whalen, R. E. and Luttge, W. G. (1971). Testosterone, androstenedione and dihydrotestosterone – effects on mating behaviour of male rats. *Hormones Behav.* 2, 117.

De Wied, D. and van Keep P. A. (eds.) (1980). *Hormones and the brain.* MTP Press, Lancaster.

Wu, F. C. W., Bancroft, J., Davidson, D. W., and Nicol, K. (1982). The behavioural effects of testosterone undecanoate in adult men with Klinefelter's syndrome: a controlled study. *Clin. Endocrinol.* 16, 489-97.

Yalom, I. D., Green, R., and Fisk, N. (1973). Prenatal exposure to female hormones. *Arch. Gen. Psychiat.* 28, 554-61.

Young, W. C. and Corner, G. W. (eds.) (1961). *Sex and internal secretions,* 3rd ed, vol. II, pp. 1387-91. Williams & Wilkins, Baltimore, MD.

5

Diagnosis of male sexual dysfunction

I. KARACAN, C. A. MOORE, C. ASLAN, AND R. L. WILLIAMS

INTRODUCTION

EVEN WITH the increased sexual openness of current times, many males suffering from impotence are still hesitant to present this complaint to a physician. None the less, Kinsey estimated in 1948 that almost one in five men became permanently impotent by the age of 60 (Kinsey, Pomeroy, and Martin 1948). Temporary impotence would seem, from anecdotal evidence alone, to be widespread as well. Until recently, conventional wisdom held that 90 per cent of cases of impotence were due to psychological, rather than physiological, causes (Cooper 1972; Hastings 1963; Masters and Johnson 1970; Strauss 1950; Wershub 1959). But a look at the means by which most cases of impotence are investigated calls the standard procedure, and thus that statistic, into question.

DIAGNOSIS OF IMPOTENCE

A comparison of the work by Keshin and Pinck (1949) with that of Compere (1978), reveals that the 'standard recommended procedure for differential diagnosis of impotence has not improved in over 30 years' (Karacan, Aslan, and Williams 1982a). Typically, the physician will perform a routine physical examination, take the patient's history, order and review standard laboratory tests for relevant physical pathology, and then examine the history of the complaint. This last is to discover signs of psychological origins, such as: rapid onset of impotence, selective or transient occurrence of impotence, or persistence of occasional masturbatory, morning, or other spontaneous erections (Simpson 1950).

Theoretically, signs of physical pathology indicate physiological roots to the complaint, whilst an onset and course consistent with the signs already mentioned will point to a psychological basis, and the presence of both indicates a mixed origin. However, in practice, the absence of clear signs or symptoms of physical problems in the routine examination leads by default to a diagnosis of psychogenic impotence (Karacan and Salis 1980).

Nocturnal penile tumescence (NPT)

We believe that improved differential diagnosis can result from monitoring of a patient's nocturnal penile tumescence (NPT), as we have undertaken in our studies. We monitored the sleep of 125 healthy males aged 3–79 years, all of whom exhibited NPT in a predictable, age-related pattern (Karacan, Hursch, Williams, and Littell 1972b; Karacan, Hursch, Williams, and Thornby

1972*c*; Hursch, Karacan and Williams 1972; Karacan, Hursch, and Williams 1972*a*; Karacan, Williams, Thornby, and Salis 1975; Karacan, Salis, Thornby, and Williams 1976). If a healthy male is expected to experience NPT, it must follow that a male with diminished or absent NPT has physiological difficulties impairing erectile capacity. Conversely, a male with normal NPT for his age who suffers impotence must then have psychological difficulties causing that impotence. These assumptions have been repeatedly substantiated in a number of studies of men with known psychological problems or disease states associated with organic erectile failure (Karacan 1982*a,b*). This still leaves the problem of identifying the possible contributory factors in the patient's complaint. The battery of tests we have developed can help to diagnose either a physiological deficit, a psychological difficulty, or a mixed psychobiological dysfunction.

That males undergo erections while asleep was first noted by Ohlmeyer and colleagues during the 1940s (Ohlmeyer, Brilmayer, and Hullstrung 1944). Karacan's study in the early 1960s recorded that 80 per cent of 237 rapid eye movement (REM) periods were accompanied by erections (Karacan 1965). That same year, Fisher's team recorded full or partial erections in 95 per cent of 86 REM periods observed in young men (Fisher, Gross, and Zuch 1965). Karacan's study, and one reported the following year (Fisher 1966), indicated that NPT and REM might be partially independent phenomena; healthy subjects deprived of REM sleep continued to exhibit NPT at those stages of the sleep cycle when REM would otherwise have occurred. Both Karacan (1965) and Fisher *et al.* (1965) noted that sexual intercourse shortly before sleep produced no changes in NPT. A series of further studies was then conducted, which have affirmed that nocturnal penile tumescence 'occurs in all normal healthy males' (Karacan 1982*a*).

Studies also showed that NPT does indeed change with age. Total NPT time per night declines from the second to the fifth decade, stabilizing at about 100 min total tumescence time. The number of REM-related episodes of NPT per night is about 4 in the third decade, dropping to 2.6 in the eighth decade. Another change in the eighth decade is that the number of full episodes decreases as the number of partial episodes rises. The length of full episodes declines from 40 min in a man's twenties to 30 min in his sixties (Karacan *et al.* 1982). Thus, researchers can now use NPT as a benchmark against which to judge the erectile capacity of a patient presenting with impotence. If a man's NPT is deficient for his years, his impotence has an origin in some physiological disturbance, such as low penile blood pressure.

Prevalence and etiology of impotence

The definition of impotence that we use is: 'an inability to obtain or sustain an erection sufficient for satisfactory conclusion of sexual intercourse'. Problems with ejaculation and reduced or absent sexual desire are not included.

The proportion of the male population suffering from erectile impotence is difficult to measure. The estimates of Kinsey and colleagues are generally cited as the most acceptable (Karacan, Salis, and Williams 1978). They are:

up to age 40, 2 per cent of men have become more or less totally and permanently impotent; by age 55, 6.7 per cent, whilst at age 60, the rate jumps to
18.4 per cent and climbs to 75 per cent by age 80 (Kinsey *et al*. 1948). Whether
impotence is becoming more prevalent is subject to dispute, but it appears
that erectile deficits, not problems with too-rapid or too-slow ejaculation or
diminution of libido, are the most frequent problems for patients seeking
treatment for sexual dysfunction (Karacan *et al*. 1978). As Shakespeare put it:
'it now remains to find the cause of this effect . . . for this effect defective comes
by cause'.

For many years, it has been conventionally accepted that 90 per cent of
impotence had psychological origins (Karacan 1982), but our evidence indicates
that this is an exaggeration. Still, some psychological states may produce impotence. Among these are: performance anxiety, depression, guilt, shame,
frustration, and negative attitudes toward sexuality, and there are others (Karacan, Williams, Derman, and Aslan 1982*b*). As for physiological roots of impotence, some conditions are known to have a high potential for impairing
erection: diabetes, alcoholism, end-stage renal disease, spinal cord injury, and
Shy-Drager syndrome (Karacan *et al*. 1982*b*). Also, vascular, neural, and neuromuscular impairment can reduce erectile capacity (Karacan 1982).

Of course, even in cases where the proximate cause of impotence is determined to be physiological, psychological difficulties may also be present. These
psychological problems may contribute to the erectile failure (i.e. mixed impotence), may result from it (i.e. secondary psychological dysfunctions, such
as reactive depression), or may not be related to it at all.

A new approach

The ancient Hebrews symbolically transferred all of their sins to a scapegoat,
whilst medieval courts had whipping boys. All too often, physicians presented
with a complaint of impotence are quick to utilize psychological factors in
such a manner. In practice, the absence of clear signs or symptoms of physical
pathology typically results in the default diagnosis of psychogenic impotence
(Karacan *et al*. 1982*a*).

The routine physical is inadequate to provide sufficient data concerning
impotence, and 'physicians often fail to perform the needed full-scale evaluation
of an impotent patient' (Karacan *et al*. 1978). The penis itself is rarely examined, either flaccid or during an attempted erection (Karacan and Ilaria
1978). Thus, the standard procedure is flawed and monitoring of nocturnal
penile tumescence is the requisite supplement. Nevertheless, categorizing a
patient's complaint as physiogenic or psychogenic is only the equivalent of
identifying an organism as animal or plant; there is still considerable identifying
work to do. Which physical deficit is causing the impotence, or which psychological problem is at the root of a patient's erectile deficiency? Our NPT monitoring and other procedures lend themselves to further isolation of the causes.

NPT MONITORING

The procedure is practical for any sleep disorders centre, but should be supplemented by developmental, sexual, marital, social, medical, psychiatric and drug histories; physical, neurological, and urological examinations; assays of testosterone and prolactin levels, a psychiatric interview, and a battery of psychological tests (Karacan *et al.* 1982*b*).

Prior to NPT monitoring, the patient is told to refrain from naps during the evaluation period and to avoid caffeine, alcohol, and non-essential drugs; these can alter sleep and NPT patterns (Karacan *et al.* 1982*b*). A preliminary general physical, including genital examination, is performed. Evidence of penile sensory deficit and pelvic or penile pain are also sought, since these may not be manifest in the form of diminished or absent NPT, but still interfere with satisfactory intercourse. Measurements of the flaccid penis are taken: length, together with tip and base circumferences. This allows selection of the proper sized NPT transducer (Karacan *et al.* 1982*b*).

The patient is monitored for three consecutive nights in a private, environmentally controlled bedroom. The first night is an adjustment period; data from this evening may be atypical due to disturbed sleep in an unfamiliar setting. The basic data are taken from the second night. On the third night, the patient is warned before bedtime that he will be awakened during his maximal erection. At that time, the erection will be photographed, the patient will be asked for his estimate of the degree and adequacy of his erection, and penile rigidity will be measured (Karacan *et al.* 1982*b*).

Degree of erection

Since in most normal men the degree of erection is represented by the increase in penile circumference, two custom-fitted mercury-filled strain gauges are placed around the patient's penis, one encircling the base and the other just below the glans. These measure changes in penile circumference during the night. Discrepancies between tip and base expansion may denote impaired penile circulation, plaque, or structural abnormality, which is why both locations are monitored. Ideally, the base will expand 1.5 to 3 times more than the tip (Karacan, *et al.* 1982*b*).

Since abnormal NPT recordings may be a result of abnormal sleep, rather than erectile deficit, electro-encephalograph (EEG) and electro-oculograph (EOG) evaluations are conducted. Bipolar, frontal, parietal, and occipital electrodes monitor EEG activity; electrodes at the outer canthi of the eyes monitor EOG activity. These also record body-movement artefacts that cause pen excursions not in fact related to erection. Methods for scoring NPT (Karacan *et al.* 1978) and EEG–EOG activity are outlined in previous reports (Rechtstaffen and Kales 1968; Williams *et al.* 1974).

Another possible contributor to unsatisfactory sexual capability is insufficient penile rigidity, which is not always measurable by penile expansion, and so a special device and procedure for monitoring this factor has been developed. When the patient is awakened for the photographing and assessment of his maximal erection on the third night, a technician presses the cap of the force-application device earlier placed on the glans, until the penis visibly bends. A constantin-foil, precision strain gauge is positioned along the dorsal midline of the penis, which automatically notes 10-degree bending. The gauge measures buckling pressures from 1 g to 1000 g; the average minimum for satisfactory vaginal intercourse is approximately 450 g (Karacan *et al.* 1982*b*).

At this time, both the patient and the technician estimate the degree of the patient's erection on a scale of 0–100 per cent. If there is a large difference between their estimates, it may be that the patient is unable to gauge his erection accurately. Indications so far are that impotent men whose NPT is organogenic are more likely to overestimate their degree of erection than are men whose impotence is psychogenic. It will require further research to determine the cause for this overestimation: actual perceptual failure, poor self-image, or deliberate mis-statement to obtain a penile prosthesis, a standard treatment for impotence having a physiological basis. A photograph provides evidence of the patient's maximum erectile capacity, disease processes, or structural defects, and also serves as a guide for a surgeon should an implant be indicated (Karacan *et al.* 1982).

Specific physiological problems

As mentioned earlier, NPT monitoring can also help to isolate the specific physiological problem evoking the impotence. During the physical examination, electrically induced bulbocavernosus (BC) relfex response latencies act as a test for the integrity of somatic segmental circuits concerned in erection. If spontaneous bulbocavernosus–ischiocavernosus activity (BCA–ICA) is detected during nocturnal erections, it may be an indication of autonomic nervous system activities. We have found that spontaneous bursts of BC–IC muscle activity precede and accompany penile circumference increases during NPT; this suggests that functional defects in these muscles may inhibit engorgement of the penis. The blood-pumping function is probably initiated above the level of the spinal cord. Thus, dissociation between BCA and NPT or NPT and REM sleep may mean a CNS dysfunction in an impotent patient (Karacan *et al.* 1982*b*).

Electrodermal activity (EDA), monitored via finger and penile electrodes, is another measure of autonomic nervous system (ANS) function. Abnormal EDA patterns are found in some men with impaired NPT and are indicative of ANS dysfunction. The electrocardiograph (ECG) is also measured during NPT monitoring. Because 'vascular problems have been discovered in more than 60 per cent of the patients presenting with impotence at our sleep disorders center', we test vascular sufficiency by comparing brachial and penile arterial pressures and also measure urethral temperature in the flaccid penis (Karacan 1982*b*). We also monitor penile pulse volume during NPT, this being measured with a photoelectric transducer over the dorsal penile artery. Occasionally, an arteriogram or cavernosogram is required to locate the exact site of vascular pathology (Karacan *et al.* 1982*b*).

Blood samples are taken and assayed to evaluate the patient's endocrine status. The drug history and collection of a urine sample for drug estimations complete the physiological evaluation. If a patient with impaired NPT consumes antihypertensive, psychoactive, or other relevant drugs on a daily basis, he is reevaluated under drug-free conditions if at all possible (Karacan *et al.* 1982*b*).

PSYCHOPATHOLOGY

The patient also undergoes a psychological/psychiatric evaluation, which is independent of the NPT monitoring. To date, there is no systematic, objective equivalent to NPT monitoring for this aspect of the evaluation. While the psychiatric interview and the psychological testing can uncover possibly relevant psychopathology, no definitive method yet exists to determine the significance of such findings to the erectile incapacity. The presence of psychological problems does not automatically prove a psychological basis for the impotence. Conversely, discovery of physiological deficits does not rule out psychological problems contributing to the ultimate result of impotence. Most impotent men show some emotional disturbance, especially in the case of long-term impotence. 'Therefore, positive evidence of psychological etiology is sought although psychogenic impotence essentially remains a default diagnosis' (Karacan *et al.* 1982*b*). A comprehensive explanation of psychonomic indicators of psychologically-produced impotence has been advanced by Beutler and colleagues (Beutler, Ware, and Karacan 1978).

The psychiatrist takes a complete history, identifying psychological, marital, or social difficulties and assessing the patient's general mental status. The interview concentrates on the timetable and exact nature of the impotence, the situations in which incapacity occurs, dynamic interaction with the partner, comparison of current sexual functioning with past sexual functioning, history of previous treatments for mental illness, and whether the patient is abusing drugs or alcohol. The psychiatrist carefully notes the temporal relationship between conditions noted in the interview and the onset or exacerbation of impotence. Family and social histories are obtained from both the patient and his sexual partner, the two being interviewed separately and, if possible, also together (Karacan *et al.* 1982*b*).

The psychological evaluation involves the patient taking an array of pencil-and-paper tests: the Shipley Institute of Living Scale, the Minnesota Multiphasic Personality Inventory (MMPI), the Loeveninger Sentence Completion Test for Men, the Derogatis Sexual Functioning Inventory, the Locke–Wallace Marital Adjustment Scale, the Profile of Mood States, the State–Trait Anxiety Inventory, and a special Reactions-to-Situations Scale which assesses performance anxiety. This battery assesses degree of psychopathology, cognitive efficiency, interpersonal expectancies and needs, current mood, sexual disturbances, and defensive style (Karacan *et al.* 1982*b*).

Many psychological states and personality traits have been linked to impotence. Unfortunately, most psychological factors in erectile deficiency are extrapolated from case studies and theoretical discussions, and in consequence experimentally derived data are unavailable (Karacan *et al.* 1982*b*).

Differential diagnosis

The final differential diagnosis is composed of the combined, independent diagnoses of each evaluator. The NPT data are emphasized in deciding whether the aetiology is psychological, physiological, or mixed. If NPT is reduced or absent, the impotence is moșt likely to be physiological in origin, whilst absent NPT indicates more severe physical dysfunction than diminished NPT. If a determination is made that the cause of the erectile deficit is physiological, an attempt is made to isolate the specific agent producing the impotence. This is done by collating the various tests and examination results (Karacan *et al.* 1982*b*).

Even this advance in diagnostic procedure is unable to specify the cause of impotence in about one in every 10 patients showing NPT diminution and no gross psychopathology. It may be that a test for some obscure cause must be added. In the future, it is to be expected that medical science will shed more light on the erectile process, especially the role of neurotransmitters; and medical technology will develop superior methods of examining autonomic nervous system defects. The latter will also involve the differentiation of central from peripheral neural deficits, and the monitoring of the interaction of psychological and physiological factors during sleep and sexual activity. In consequence, it is reasonable to expect a shrinking, perhaps an elimination of this statistic (Karacan *et al.* 1982*b*).

EXPERIMENTAL RESULTS

Having utilized NPT monitoring in over several thousand cases of impotence, our sleep disorders centre noted diminished or absent nocturnal penile tumescence in over 64 per cent. While this is somewhat biased, since most of our patients were being screened for implantation of a penile prosthesis, it matches results from six other centres performing NPT evaluations in cases of impotence; their incidence of NPT deficits was 66 per cent (Karacan 1982).

Thus, rather than the possibility of a physiological aetiology being casually dismissable, it becomes of equal importance when a physician is presented with a complaint of impotence. The incidence is 'too large for any responsible, knowledgeable physician to ignore' (Karacan and Ilaria 1978). Therefore, we concluded that the monitoring of NPT should be performed in the evaluation of all males complaining of impotence (Karacan and Ilaria 1978). Of course, even the discovery of a biological basis for a case of impotence should not preclude an attempt to uncover psychological problems; aetiology can be mixed. The tests we have included in our arsenal have shown value in isolating specific problems. For example, we have identified vascular insufficiency as the reason for erectile deficiency in more than 60 per cent of the men whose monitoring revealed reduced or absent NPT (Karacan 1982). Other tests have helped to locate the aetiology of impotence in many other cases.

Of course, once a cause has been identified, the patient can be referred for treatment. This may be psychotherapy, vascular surgery, endocrine treatment, or a penile prosthesis. The important fact is that now we have a way of knowing, in most cases, what to recommend.

Other new techniques

A portable NPT monitor has been developed, which may make NPT monitoring more easily available. Sleep EEG and rigidity measurements should be incorporated into the portable system so that reliability and validity are not compromised.

A recently developed technique, the stamp method of measuring NPT, consists of encircling the flaccid penis with postage stamps from a roll and sticking the two end stamps together. It is assumed that if they break during the night, the subject has good erectile function. This is not however an acceptable method of evaluating erectile capacity. Problems are: (1) breaking of stamps due to movement rather than erection; (2) weakening and premature breakage due to moisture; (3) slippage of stamps; (4) occasional lack of breakage even with full erection, causing pain and hypoxia of the penis; and (5) inability to determine duration, conformation, and rigidity of the penis, all of which are important to sexual functioning.

Two other methods of assessing erectile function are the showing of erotic films and/or masturbation. These can be helpful, and are inexpensive when the patient has an erection which is clearly of sufficient size, duration, and rigidity. But negative results, or partial or brief erections, are inconclusive. Some men who are potent do not achieve erections under laboratory conditions. Also, some patients may find erotic films or masturbation in the laboratory distasteful or offensive.

Improving monitoring

An area of possible improvement is the use of NPT observation in investigating the mechanism of erection and impotence (Karacan *et al*. 1978). We have many completed and ongoing studies in which NPT monitoring is used to examine drug and disease effects on erectile capacity.

Improvements in the monitoring procedure are always to be desired. For one thing, we continue to search for exceptions to the apparently general rule that abnormalities in NPT are reliable indicators of organic involvement in impotence. A few potential exceptions have already been found: for example, isolated penile sensory deficit. This does not impede NPT, since NPT is independent of external stimulation, but it would impair a sexual erection (Karacan 1982). However, we test for such a deficit. Another rarely seen example is 'gluteal steal syndrome', in which blood from the penile circulation is shunted to gluteal muscles during exercise, when the gluteal circulation is impaired. A patient with the syndrome might be able to have normal erections during sleep, but during intercourse the shunting might take place. The patients have a history of buttock pain on exercise and ability to obtain an erection at rest, but inability to maintain it during exercise. We find decreased penile blood pressure after pelvic exercise.

Also, methodological modifications are needed to develop a more sensitive means of (1) examining local and central autonomic nervous system dysfunction, (2) differentiating central from peripheral neural deficits, and (3) monitoring the interaction of psychological variables with physiological processes during sleep and sexual activity (Karacan *et al.* 1982*a*). Of course, improvements in the equipment are needed. One such advance would be developments, already underway, in computer technology associated with the transducer that measures rigidity (Karacan *et al.* 1982*a*).

CONCLUSIONS

Let us delineate what we have learned in our research:

(1) Most impotent men with a high probability of organogenic impotence have reduced or absent NPT.

(2) Most impotent men with a low probability of organogenic impotence have normal NPT.

(3) Impotent men with diminished or absent NPT benefit from correction of the physiological problems leading to their impotence. In the case of impaired genital circulation, vascular surgery enhances erectile capacity.

(4) Men with diminished NPT do not have their erectile functioning improved by psychological assistance.

(5) Conversely, impotent men with normal NPT do not have their waking erectile capability enhanced by medical treatment, but often have improved erectile capacity following psychological assistance.

(6) General or acute psychological factors do not significantly inhibit NPT.

(7) A subject's level or recency of sexual activity does not affect NPT (Karacan *et al.* 1982*a*).

'Tomorrow', Scarlett O'Hara told us, 'is another day'. It promises to be an even better day for men suffering from impotence, because the likelihood is that improvements and enhancements in monitoring nocturnal penile tumescence will make it easier to locate the source of their complaints.

References

Beutler, L. W., Ware, C., and Karacan, I. (1978). Psychological assessment of the sexually impotent male. In *Sleep disorders: diagnosis and treatment* (eds. R. L. Williams and I. Karacan), pp. 383-94. John Wiley, New York.

Compere, J. S. (1978). Office recognition and management of erectile dysfunction. *Am. Fam. Phys.* **17**, 186-90.

Cooper, A. J. (1972). The causes and management of impotence. *Postgrad. Med. J.* **48**, 548-52.

Fisher, C. (1966). Dreaming and sexuality. In *Psychoanalysis – a general psychology. Essays in honor of Heinz Hartmann* (eds. R. M. Loewenstein, L. M. Newman, M. Schur, and A. J. Solnit) pp. 537-69. International Universities Press, New York.

–– Gross, J., and Zuch, J. (1965). Cycle of penile erection synchronous with dreaming (REM) sleep. *Arch. Gen. Psychiat.* **12**, 29-45.

Hastings, D. W. (1963). *Impotence and frigidity*, p. 45. Little, Brown, Boston.

Hursch, C. J., Karacan, I., and Williams, R. L. (1972). Some characteristics of nocturnal penile tumescence in early middle-aged males. *Comp. Psychiat.* **13**, 539-48.

Karacan, I. (1965). The effect of exciting presleep events on dream reporting and penile erections during sleep. Unpublished doctoral dissertation, Downstate Medical Center, State University of New York.

—— (1982*a*). Evaluation of nocturnal penile tumescence and impotence. In *Sleeping and waking disorders: indications and techniques* (ed. C. Guilleminault), p. 345. Addison-Wesley, Menlo Park, Ca.

—— (1982*b*). Nocturnal penile tumescence as a biologic marker in assessing erectile dysfunction. *Psychosomatics* 23 (4).

—— and Ilaria, R. L. (1978). Nocturnal penile tumescence (NPT): The phenomenon and its role in the diagnosis of impotence. *Sexual. Disabil.* 1, 260-71.

—— and Salis, P. J. (1980). Diagnosis and treatment of erectile impotence. *Psychiat. Clin. N.Am.* 3, 97-111.

—— Aslan, C., and Williams, R. L. (1982*a*). Diagnostic evaluation of male impotence: Problems and promises. In *Phenomenology and treatment of psychosexual disorders* (ed. W. E. Fann, I. Karacan, A. D. Pokorny, and R. L. Williams). Spectrum, New York.

—— Hursch, C. J., and Williams, R. L. (1972*a*). Some characteristics of nocturnal penile tumescence in elderly males. *J. Gerontol.* 27, 39-45.

—— —— and Littell, R. C. (1972*b*). Some characteristics of nocturnal penile tumescence during puberty. *Pediatr. Res.* 6, 529-37.

—— —— —— and Thornby, J. I. (1972*c*). Some characteristics of nocturnal penile tumescence in young adults. *Arch. Gen. Psychiat.* 26, 351-6.

—— Salis, P. J., and Williams, R. L. (1978). The role of the sleep laboratory in diagnosis and treatment of impotence. In *Sleep disorders: diagnosis and treatment* (eds. R. L. Williams and I. Karacan), pp. 353-82. John Wiley, New York.

—— —— Thornby, J. I., and Williams, R. L. (1976). The ontogeny of nocturnal penile tumescence. *Waking and Sleeping* 1, 27-44.

—— Scott, F. B., Hartse, K., Williams, R. L., and Takanami, M. (in press). Incidence of erectile dysfunction in the sleep disorders center. In *Long-term evolution and natural history of sleep disorders* (eds. C. Guilleminault and E. Lugaresi). Raven Press, New York.

—— Williams, R. L., Derman, S., and Aslan, C. (1982*b*). Impaired, sleep-related penile tumescence in the diagnosis of impotence. In *Eating, sleeping, and sexuality: treatment of disorders in basic life functions* (ed. M. R. Zales), pp. 186-99. Brunner-Mazel, New York.

—— —— Thornby, J. I., and Salis, P. J. (1975). Sleep related penile tumescence as a function of age. *Am. J. Psychiat.* 132, 932-7.

Keshin, J. G., and Pinck, B. D. (1949). Impotentia. *N.Y. State J. Med.* 49, 269-72.

Kinsey, A. C., Pomeroy, A. B., and Martin, C. E. (1948). *Sexual behavior in the human male*, p. 236. Saunders, Philadelphia.

Masters, W. H. and Johnson, V. E. (1970). *Human sexual inadequacy*. Little, Brown, Boston.

Ohlmeyer, P., Brilmayer, H., and Hullstrung, H. (1944). Periodisch organge im Schlaf. *Pfleugers Arch.* 248, 559-60.

Rechtschaffen, A., and Kales, A. (1968). *A manual of standardized terminology, techniques and scoring system for sleep stages of human subjects.* U.S. Government Printing Office, Washington, DC.

Simpson, S. L. (1950). Impotence. *Br. Med. J.* 1, 692-7.

Strauss, E. B. (1950). Impotence from the psychiatric standpoint. *Br. Med. J.* 1, 697-9.

Wershub, L. P. (1959). *Sexual impotence in the male*, pp. 27, 29. Charles C. Thomas, Springfield, Il.

Williams, R. L., Karacan, I., and Hursch, C. J. (1974). *Electroencephalography (EEG) of human sleep: Clinical applications.* John Wiley, New York.

Editorial Assistant on this chapter was Jeff Daiell.

Sex in the community

6

Sexual anxieties and their treatment

ALEX COMFORT

INTRODUCTION

ANXIETIES focused on sexuality are of two kinds; fundamental or human, and endemic. Acceptability, gender, and self-image are potential sources of worry for the unself-assured in all cultures; sexuality *per se* has been made a particular focus of anxiety in our own. 'Sexual anxiety' in the doctor's office accordingly comes in three sizes, with overlap between the psychodynamics involved. The first consists of the general consequences of low self-esteem, which may be focused on body image, on potency, and on gender, and may be expressed in dysfunction, acting-out, or both. Next comes acquired guilt, discomfort, and fear, attached to sexuality in general or to particular manifestations such as masturbation. Finally, there are situational and specific anxieties; about sexual preferences, sexual symptoms such as premature ejaculation or anorgasmia, or complications in a particular marital or sociosexual relationship.

THE APPROACH TO THE PROBLEM

The approach of the informed physician is now that whichever of these presentations occupies the foreground of the complaint, the others are present in the background, so that direct attack on a symptom, even if it works, will leave both patient and physician out of their depth and open a can of worms which would have been much better left to 'those whose business it is'.

Overzealous symptomatic counselling can certainly do this; on the other hand the family doctor is, with a modicum of judgement, an excellent source of sex counselling, provided that he has a psychiatric 'green thumb', and can read from non-verbal signals how far down in the patient and the patient's relationship the problem actually goes. It needs to be repeated that although sexual problems may have profound psychodynamic roots, they may equally arise from specific physical, commonsense, or pharmacological origins which can be removed in short order. Confronted with a complaint of 'ejaculatory incompetence', for example, one may indeed be seeing a manifestation of hostility to the spouse, or the patient may be on an antihypertensive, an antidepressant, or some other medication known to delay or abolish the ejaculatory reflex. On the other hand, he may be one of the relatively numerous males who react to fatigue, age, or preoccupation, by non-ejaculation rather than impotency. The test of the physician is in the correctness of his guess after a proper history and an interview with both partners.

SOCIAL ANXIETIES

Aside from general low self-esteem or free-floating anxiety about the propriety and worthiness of sexual feelings and behaviours (which can be just as present in the ostensibly 'liberated' and unconventional as in hard-line Puritans), there are a number of common problems involving sexual anxiety as an explicit presentation. The commonest of these is unease over a particular sexual behaviour, often masturbation, oral intercourse, or a minor fetish, followed by misunderstanding, or folklore-based misinformation, about the normal physiology of sex and the normal changes which occur with age, stress, and the like. Next come gender anxieties, and finally anxieties relating to body image. Excluded from this list are the specific sexual symptomatologies such as impotence, premature ejaculation, and anorgasmia, because these both generate anxiety and can result from, or be maintained by, anxiety. They have accordingly to be evaluated on an individual basis.

Generalized anxieties are focussed on sexuality by a wealth of misinformation available from books, parents, peers, physicians, and religious teachers. The approved model for dealing with them in the first instance is probably still educational rather than medical and this involves moving through permission, limited information, special information, and finally therapy if required.

PHARMACOLOGY AND SEX

Since some sexual anxiety arises in specific physical disorders, medication may obviously have a place in this phase of therapy, but in general the psychopharmacology of sexual anxiety is negative, not positive. It consists, in the main, in the removal of medications which are incidentally affecting sexual function, including alcohol, and is a far commoner requirement than the prescription of specific drug therapy.

Adverse drug effects

The most frequent pharmacological causes of sexual dysfunction in males are antihypertensive drugs, antidepressants, tranquillizers and, of course, alcohol. The inhibitory effects of reserpine and methyldopa are familiar, as evidenced by the degree of non-compliance by the patient in drug taking, but about 7 per cent of males on thiazides and a small proportion on propranolol (Knarr 1976) develop drug-induced impotency or failure of ejaculation. Most tricyclics tend, if they affect sexuality, to inhibit ejaculation. So do mono-amine oxidase inhibitors (MAOI), which also provide one of the few documented examples of drug interference with response in women, a topic grossly neglected so far by male-oriented physicians (Lesko, Stotland, and Taylor-Segraves 1982). Both female anorgasmia and male impotency are reported with amoxepin (Schwarcz 1982), which can also cause painful ejaculation (Kulik and Wilbur 1982). Where this problem with antidepressants gives rise to non-compliance, it can often be relieved without stopping the drug, either by dose titration, or in some instances by bethanecol.

Numerous other medications can trigger sexual dysfunction, which may be varied, idiosyncratic, and unreported in the literature, and this cause should always be excluded before embarking on interpretative psychotherapy. Some pharmacological traps for the wouldbe psychoanalyst are less obvious but manifest to commonsense, such as the prescription of oestrogen, with consequent overlubrication, to a wife whose husband is experiencing the normal age-dependent need for increased friction in intercourse.

Major tranquillizers

Major tranquillizers affect sexuality irregularly; they may inhibit erection, ejaculation, both, or neither, in different patients (Kotin, Wilbert, Verburg, and Soldinger 1976). This wide variation is typical of many drugs used in the relief of mental symptoms, where sexual function develops with associated anxiety. Under these circumstances, one must, as it were, trade off the effects of the underlying disorder, its psychodynamic relation to sexuality if it has one, the effects of medication on function, and the effects of dysfunction in reviving sexually-oriented anxiety.

In the case of alcohol, similar considerations apply, but the medication is self-administered. The depressed subject may be both dysfunctional and sexually anxious, and may add alcoholic inhibition of erection and androgen production to the mixture. Occasional or 'social' alcohol consumption can trigger situational impotence, and set off a functionally-autonomous cycle of failure–performance anxiety–more failure, in consequence of which the patient then presents for treatment. The same cycle can be initiated by medication unrelated to anxiety (clofibrate provided an unexpected example). The sexual side-effect may not be reported to the physician unless sought.

I mention these side-effects in the context of this chapter because dysfunctions always lead to anxiety, and can inflame pre-existing anxiety in those with personality problems. The effect is compounded if, for example, an antihypertensive drug is ordered because the doctor has made the patient anxious about hypertension. Another example is the antidepressant prescribed to reduce anxiety secondary to a free-standing depression, which itself is likely to interfere with libido.

IATROGENIC ANXIETIES

Another group of iatrogenic anxieties arise in cardiac and stroke patients who fantasize that exertion exposes them to the risk of sudden death. Since sexuality is by atavistic consent a morally dangerous activity, sex becomes the focus of fear that it may be visited by sudden death, and the illness used as an excuse to avoid it. These associations are not often conscious, and it is a function of proper rehabilitation to head them off by explicit permission, together with antianginal drugs to be taken before coitus. Even the complaint of post-prostatectomy dysfunction is quite commonly the realization of a fear which has not been acknowledged, rather than a consequence of surgery.

The role of misinformation

Acute and chronic sexual anxiety due to idiotic advice, which may come from peers and neighbours, but also, unfortunately, from the physician, is still seen.

This is so especially if the patient musunderstands what is being said, although this is becoming less common with the growth of public information. Misinformation about, for example, masturbation, given 60 or 70 years ago, may continue to smoulder in elderly subjects. Moreover a new category of anxiogenic malinstruction has grown up with the advent of 'try-anything' or 'liberated' sexual therapists. Those who were formerly made anxious by doctors over normal sexual practices, may now be made anxious if they have *not* 'tried everything' or achieved unrealistic levels of arousal. It is specially evident in geriatric medicine that where there is sexual anxiety there has nearly always been contributory misinformation, but a forecast of the future only suggests that the misinformation of tomorrow will be different, not that patients will be correctly informed of the facts.

LIMITATIONS OF PSYCHOPHARMACOLOGY

Where anxiety is deep seated, even if it is attached to a single concern such as masturbation, homosexual drives, or body image, there is no specific need for medication. Patients may still receive it, however, because the physician is ill at ease about undertaking psychotherapy. Often the patient is persistent, and repeated discourse about his small penis, her lack of satisfaction, or the demoralizing character of their normal-range homosexual responses, can assume the mantle of a delusional state, or at least an intractable one. The use of minor tranquillizers and sedatives in psychiatry is limited to tiding-over crisis reactions. They have precious little application in sex counselling, since even the individual whose dysfunction comes from worrying about the possibility of dysfunction, rarely does better when sedated. Some cases of premature ejaculation are a possible exception to this, for in such cases the slowing-down effects of a small dose of a sedative tricyclic may dismiss the problem. In general, at the point where educative reassurance has failed and the temptation to sedate arises, the patient should be referred to a psychiatric or a sexual dysfunction clinic.

Anxiety and impotence

Anxious patients with impotency or anorgasmia have a knack of making the doctor anxious too. The temptation to 'try androgens', on the basis that they may act as a placebo if for no other reason, should be resisted. The doctor should adopt the initial measures including education and reassurance, and a review of drugs and alcohol. Then, there is John Hunter's celebrated cure, which was to continue sleeping with the partner but on no account to have intercourse with her for a month, whereupon 'the fear of performance being removed, the animal spirits reassert themselves'. If these measures fail, the choice is between referral and undertaking proper investigation, including sleep plethysmography, to establish whether the problem is psychogenic or physical. Many patients have received extensive counselling and adjuration to 'get in touch with their bodies', in the presence of unrecognized early diabetes or a prolactinoma (Spark, White, and Connolly 1980). A few cases are improved by androgen (Davidson, Camargo, and Smith 1979), but if we exclude evidently androgen-deficient individuals, these are usually older males in poor physical condition, and the gain is as much an effect of increased wellbeing as of resexualization.

Indications for drug therapy

In sum, the only sexually-oriented anxieties which respond to psychopharmacology, are those which are incidental symptoms of a treatable or modifiable mental illness such as affective disorder or schizophrenia. The therapy is that of the disease itself, to be administered with due care that the symptom is not aggravated by the drug with consequent triggering of a new round of sexual anxiety.

I know of only two exceptions to this approach. One is the relatively rare case, in ordinary practice, of the individual whose anxiety is justified because his sexual peculiarity is antisocial, such as compulsive paedophilia or exhibitionism. Here one can secure some respite for all parties concerned by using an anti-androgen (see Chapter 13). Cyproterone has the advantage of suppressing fantasy more than it suppresses routine intercourse, and can sometimes be titrated to normalize rather than castrate the patient. Patients sometimes ask intelligently whether the offending impulse can be turned off, or down, and this request may in fact indicate the line of treatment.

The other is the extraordinary condition of paroxysmal sexual anxiety known as koro, formerly believed to be an unfortunate cultural creation of the Chinese, but now reported with increasing frequency in Europeans (Barrett 1978; Constable 1979). This is characterized by the sudden onset of acute anxiety accompanied by a sensation of shrinking in the genitalia, which seem about to disappear. In spite of the psychoanalytic temptations which this odd experience offers, there is some ground for thinking that what is involved is a sympathetic 'storm' of some kind, with contraction of the cremasters. Amputees often respond to the sound of an unexpected gunshot with a sudden twinge in the stump, and this will also produce sensations referred to the genitalia in many normal males, as part of the syndrome of being 'made to jump'. Cases of koro are rare indeed in clinical practice, but in the event of seeing such a case, we might do well to look for cardiac causes (floppy mitral valve) and to attempt to prevent recurrence with a beta-blocker, if no such cause was found.

Aside from the treatment of sexual anxiety, all psychopharmacologists would welcome a certain means of overriding its effects in impotency. The fact that we know many drugs which interfere with sexual function and none which trigger it reliably, is an indication of the psychophysiological complexity of the normal sexual response, which involves central, spinal, vascular, sympathetic, and parasympathetic elements. In fact, the most probable coordinated mediator of erectile function is a distinct substance, the vasoactive intestinal peptide (Polak 1981; Wagner, Bro-Rasmussen, Willis, and Nielsen 1982), for which special receptors exist in erectile tissue. Whether this mechanism will provide ways of short-circuiting the dysfunctional effects of anxiety is unclear. The association of potency with high dominance and lack of anxiety is probably finely woven as an adaptive mechanism in primate evolution, and there is probably no aphrodisiac active at a peripheral level, which central influences cannot override.

Drugs in the female

The evident concentration in the foregoing on the male patient is not a consequence of auctorial insensitivity, for women are probably more frequently and indiscriminately medicated than men, if they complain of sexual problems. It results from a culpable lack of interest in the sexual side-effects of medication on women. We have data for only a few drugs as to how they affect response time, lubrication, orgasm, and other aspects of sexual function. Not even the benzodiazepine-sodden clientele of some geographic regions have asked whether their prescriptions, and their visits to the 'sex therapist', may not be interrelated. Nor has anyone investigated such a relationship. The action of some psychoactive drugs in releasing prolactin may be an important contributor to female dysfunction, but if it is we have no data on it. This large neglected area of psychopharmacology can only be opened up by the inclusion of proper routine sex histories in the standard examination.

Just as sexual dysfunction and sexual anxiety in males have a chicken and egg relationship, which can be demonstrated if the dysfunction is systematically investigated and relieved, so not a few longtime female customers of exhortatory sex therapists have become enthusiastically orgasmic on small doses of bromocryptine. Ordinary medicine and psychodynamics can each enable us to deal properly with some cases of sexual anxiety and the *tertium quid* is judgement, which will dictate the proper proportion of each in the management plan.

CONCLUSIONS

Anxieties over matters sexual are of considerable importance in both males and females and should be systematically approached by the physician or sex counsellor. Although the approved model for treatment is, in the first instance, educational rather than medical, psychopharmacology does have a precise although limited role in treatment.

It is important to exclude psychotropic medication as a cause of both sexual anxieties and dysfunction, and it is important also to consider iatrogenic anxieties induced in patients with physical disorders, by well-meaning advisers. Drugs may be particularly indicated in cases of anti-social sexual behaviour and, in the rare case of koro a β-blocking drug may be specifically indicated. Ordinary medical principles, a knowledge of psychodynamics, and fine clinical judgement will enable the physician to decide upon the best means of treating anxieties associated with sexual functions.

References

Barrett, K. (1978). Koro in a Londoner. *Lancet* ii, 1319.
Constable, P. J. (1979). Koro in Hertfordshire. *Lancet* i, 163.
Davidson, J. M., Camargo, C. A., and Smith, E. R. (1979). Effects of androgen on sexual behavior in hypogonadal men. *J. Clin. Endocrinol. Metab.* **48**, 955–8.
Knarr, J. W. (1976). Impotence from propranolol? *Ann Int. Med.* **85**, 259.

Kotin, J., Wilbert, D. E., Verburg, D., and Soldinger, S. M. (1976). Thioridazine and sexual dysfunction. *Am. J. Psychiat.* **133**, 82–4.

Kulik, F. A. and Wilbur, R. (1982). Case report of painful ejaculation as a side-effect of amoxapine. *Am.J. Psychiat.* **139**, 234–5.

Lesko, L. M., Stotland, N. L., and Taylor-Segraves, R. (1982). Three cases of female anorgasmia associated with MAOI's. *Am. J. Psychiat.* **139**, 1353–4.

Polak, J. M., Mina, S., Gu, J., and Bloom, S. R. (1981). Vipergic nerves in the penis. *Lancet* ii, 217–19.

Schwarcz, G. (1982). Case report of inhibition of ejaculation and retrograde ejaculation as side effects of amoxapine. *Am. J. Psychiat.* **139**, 233.

Spark, R. F., White, R. A., and Connolly, P. B. (1980). Impotence is not always psychogenic. *J. Am. Med. Ass.* **243**, 750–6.

Wagner, G., Bro-Rasmussen, F., Willis, E. A., and Niesen, M. H. (1982). New theory of the mechanism of erection involving hitherto undescribed vessels. *Lancet* i, 416–18.

7

Sexuality in old age, illness, and disability

DOMEENA C. RENSHAW

INTRODUCTION

AT WHAT AGE do men and women burn out sexually? One indignant 'Louisiana Gentleman', well past 70 years, wrote in to a popular newspaper columnist: "A man stops being sexual only when he is officially declared dead". The gentleman insisted that, with the proper stimulation, a man or woman at any age may be aroused and that sex was healthy for the heart, lungs, and blood circulation. After a nationally televised program, an 83-year-old woman wrote a delightful letter to me requesting a reading list, because she wanted to have "an organism before I die". After signing off she added: "P.S., I looked it up in Webster's dictionary. I guess they call it an orgasm these days".

How can wrinkles, arthritis, grey hair, sagging tissues, prostatectomy, hysterectomy, coronary, stroke, cancer, hypertension, diabetes, multiple sclerosis, etc. go along with being sexual. Does not society say sex is for the young, the beautiful, and the healthy? Does not society insist that ageing is a season of losses, most of all, of losing sexual desire? Are the old and the disabled not 'expected' to be sexually inactive? But are they? Indeed not. Sexual feelings, for many elderly men and women in sickness and in health, endure and continue into late age, despite all of the family and cultural negatives. Despite some changes in sexual performance with ageing and illness, desire, interest, and sexual activity continue, as does the search for an interested and/or interesting partner (Busse and Pfeiffer 1977; Butler 1975; Butler and Lewis 1977; Wasow and Loeb 1978).

EFFECTS OF AGEING

Certainly, as mentioned, there may be some slowing of sexual responses (rather than feelings) due to vascular, hormonal, mobility, or other physical factors of illness and ageing, but not necessarily cessation of sexual fantasy or interest. The more active generally and sexually an individual was as a young person, the more active and sexual they will continue to be. The youthful impulsivity of a sexual encounter, with its urgency of genital penetration, power, and procreation may wane; but the senior becomes more sexually experienced, more in control of ejaculation or orgasm, and may engage and savour leisurely foreplay and afterplay. Some are able to incorporate new sexual knowledge and with this cognitive help discard ancient taboos and sexual guilts. This may allow them to be flexible and use coital alternatives, deriving sexual joy from sensual pleasuring and emotional closeness without intercourse, yet enhancing intimacy.

Psychological factors

Recognition of the importance of sexuality in the lives of the elderly is long overdue. Many are themselves embarrassed by their desires and they need the encouragement of the physician to enable them to express their views honestly, and then reveal their problems. It is up to the physician to explain that these can be discussed no matter how old the patient. Their questions may contain the same ignorance as those of teenagers and others. Few, despite the 'sex revolution' have had a good sex education, which is a major aspect of sex therapy; very possible from a physician who is a trusted authority.

The popular view of sex therapy clinics is that they deal with the malfunctions of the young and, possibly, the middle-aged. A careful study of the ages of those treated at sex clinics shows how eager older people are to seek aid once they realize that it is available to them. The oldest couple treated at the Masters–Johnson Institute of Reproductive Biology in St. Louis, Missouri, was an 88-year-old woman and her 93-year-old husband. Among the couples treated at the Loyola of Chicago Sex Clinic, 20 per cent were over 50 and 20 per cent of those were over 65; the oldest was a 77-year-old woman and her 83-year-old husband. Each year more and more older patients request treatment.

Certainly, despite cosmetic surgery and vitamins, ageing does change sexual as well as all other functions. The physician can explain that although the intensity of the orgasmic response may diminish, due to the reality of decreased muscle strength and vascularity, subjective desire, enjoyment, and satisfaction can be as intense or even greater than in youth.

Sexual changes after fifty

For women these are: (a) reduced vaginal lubrication (oestrogen responsive) and (b) increased laxity of the vagina (reduced connective tissue elasticity). For men, they are: (a) delayed and/or partial (reduced height) erections (arteriosclerosis and reduced connective tissue elasticity); (b) reduced fluid and force of ejaculation; (c) plateau phase prolonged (sustained erection); (d) more rapid detumescence post-orgasm, and (e) increased refractory period before the next erection–ejaculation cycle (Masters and Johnson 1970).

At the National Gerontology Research Center, Baltimore, careful studies on the relationship of testosterone luteinizing hormone, follicle stimulating hormone, and sexual activity have been in process for some years. What emerges is that the more sexually active the male, the higher his testosterone levels as if the sex activity itself is a stimulus to increased hormone secretion (Harman and Tsitouras 1980; Tsitouras 1982). More investigation is needed, particularly since high alcohol consumption was noted in the 'low' sex activity control group. Alcohol has sedative properties on the cortex besides effectively lowering testosterone.

Longitudinal studies undertaken at Duke University showed that 70 per cent of 68-year-old and 25 per cent of octogenarian men regularly had intercourse, as did the majority of women in their 70s if they had an active partner (Busse and Pfeiffer 1977). The availability of a partner determined the sexual activity. The physician should be particularly sensitive to the problems that the single state produces for the solitary older woman and also for the wife of an impotent man (Renshaw 1981*a*). Her normal sexual feelings and behaviour may cause painful guilt feelings, whilst insecurity or self-blame may keep a widow from an active sexual search. The restricted available male peer partner pool is real and may further discourage her. She may suffer needless guilt about masturbation or the use of a vibrator to release her natural sexual tensions. The physician can help her by pointing out that sexual arousal is normal and healthy (Renshaw 1981*b*).

Diagnostic problems

Some patients may complain of constipation or vague headache, when they really want to ask: 'Is it normal to have sexual feelings at 60?'. A laxative or a mild tranquillizer for the manifest rather than actual presenting complaint, will, therefore, bring only temporary relief. When issuing a prescription, the alert physician will take an extra 10 minutes to inquire about social activities, loneliness, and sexual feelings, to prevent a return with the same unexpressed problem.

The crucial questions should be casual, routine, and open-ended: 'How do you handle your sexual feelings?' for example. At this point, the physician should be prepared to provide accurate medical and sexual information about the range of normal function from youth to old age. Such a discussion must be approached with sensitivity toward the patient's personal value system and sexual attitudes. In our culture, there may also be a feeling of shame about an ageing body. The doctor can advise older patients about diet and skin care, and reassure them about their sexual capabilities.

There are many practical and simple ways to assist older couples with sexual problems. Consider the woman whose 53-year-old husband experiences only a partial erection for the first time and he panics. Impotence might follow, not because he is ageing but as a result of his anxiety; but this is emotional impotence based on misinformation. If his wife has no greater knowledge, she may, out of compassion, avoid him sexually; 'not to be in bed and upset him because he cannot . . .'. The couple then has no loving contact at all, which may aggravate the distress of both and lead to both physical and needless emotional distance. They should be told that with prolonged foreplay and simple caressing, totally and genitally, the husband can build up to a functional erection which, although of reduced height, often lasts longer than when he was younger. Therefore, their sexual exchange may actually be enhanced.

Women who have reduced lubrication after the age of 50, or following a total hysterectomy, may benefit from hormones, systemic or in a cream, or from generous application of a vaginal lubricant such as mineral oil jelly. Sexually active women are less likely to become dry. For both sexes, the old adage still applies: 'If you don't use it, you'll lose it' (McConnell and Anderson 1980; Renshaw 1979*a*).

ARTHRITIS AND SEX

There have been no systematic, large-scale studies of the prevalence of sexual difficulties among the millions of persons afflicted with various forms of arthritis.

In a small study of 58 patients with juvenile rheumatoid arthritis, two thirds reported limitation of sexual activity because of pain, fatigue, or position problems (Engleman and Silverman 1979). Yet, having grown up with arthritis, they had adapted to it and felt no different from their peers in regard to sexual activity. Some members of the group did request sex counselling and wished that they had had this at an earlier age.

Age at onset

A patient's social life and dating and mating pattern are strongly affected by the age at onset of arthritis. A teenager's need to look like his or her peers and to associate with them, is part of the developmental process. Activity, especially participation and competition in sports and, for example, learning the latest dance steps, is often essential for the adolescent's self-perception. For one with juvenile rheumatoid arthritis, inability to share in these activities may result in social withdrawal and self-pity, and perhaps sublimation via more solitary intellectual activities. The consequent reduction in potential peer partners means that dating and the eventual choice of a lifelong partner may be limited to other disabled peers.

The fear of ridicule or pity can be impediments to an adolescent's healthy social life. Occasionally, a young arthritic's denial of illness may take the form of promiscuity to prove his or her value, at least in the area of sex. Promiscuity may also be a misguided trade-off, whereby the patient offers sex as a means of obtaining a sense of closeness and the enjoyment of being held and loved. All of the attendant complications that may be encountered, the possibilities of pregnancy, abandonment, and venereal disease make maturation that much more difficult for an arthritic teenager.

Marital relations

The arthritic patient who is already married may find the relationship strained because of physical disability. 'For better or for worse' can become dramatically and painfully real. With some couples, the affected spouse becomes overdependent, which can result in conflict or rejection, or even divorce. Some marital partners abhor illness and disability; they may consider them to constitute a personal weakness, or feel ashamed socially, and thus be unable to understand or support the ill spouse. They may avoid sexual relations with the arthritic spouse, perhaps fearing contagion or that they may inflict pain with intercourse. A man may lose his erection if his wife cries out in pain when he mounts, and he may not again approach her sexually, which makes her feel undesirable and isolated.

If the arthritic spouse gets joint pain when the normal partner moves in bed, the couple may begin sleeping apart. They then both lose the needed nightly caressing, touching, affection, and emotional support. This couple may still relate to one another during times of acute crisis throughout the long-term course of the illness, but such sporadic attention may be insufficient to sustain a happy relationship. Because arthritis may be characterized by acute exacerbations alternating with remissions, an insensitive spouse may think the patient is exaggerating the suffering and may make an accusation of faking or hypochondriasis. This kind of personal stress may create even more problems than the arthritis itself, preventing closeness, affection, and sexual exchange.

Psycho-sexual problems

Any physician who cares for an arthritic patient should be on the alert for signs and expressions of hopelessness and helplessness regarding the illness, and for possible clinical depression. Remember that depression reduces all of the appetites; for food, sleep, sex, and life. With or without arthritis, the patient who exhibits depression is in need of immediate and vigorous treatment with antidepressant medication and, possibly, psychotherapy.

If the onset of arthritis results in impotence or loss of orgasmic potential, are these problems due to pain, medications, or mechanical position difficulties? They may be caused by other issues such as anxiety, depression, or resentment or anger between the partners. An able-bodied spouse may feel cheated, or chained to a spouse 'crippled' by arthritis. He or she may cope with the overall life stress of this debilitating illness, through alcohol, deliberate control of sexual expression, or extramarital affairs, but these behaviours may also have been used before the illness.

Prescribed and over-the-counter medications that arthritic patients may take, such as analgesics, muscle relaxants, hypnotics, tranquillizers, anti-depressants, anti-inflammatory drugs, and corticosteroids, can cause a variety of physical as well as specifically chemical sexual side-effects. All or any of these drugs may reduce general and genital sensations, thus lowering sexual pleasure. Analgesic medications may reduce libido, whilst steroids may be associated with weight gain, rounding of the face and neck, gastritis, hypertension, and water retention. Emotional distress may ensue because of altered physical appearance, but steroids may also promote a sense of well-being, improved mobility, and euphoria. Some hypnotics and tranquillizers cause partial erections, delayed ejaculations, or impotence.

If arthritis results in limitation of movement or pain when sore joints are touched, it may impede sexual performance, but it rarely reduces the *desire* for loving contact and sexual exchange between concerned and caring partners. However, emotional conflict and interactional problems between partners may indeed be manifested as a libido problem, as well as mechanical sexual dysfunction. Both in relation to general movement as well as to sexual activity, the more active they are the better.

Management

Taking a sexual history should be routine in caring for a patient with arthritis. If a teenager has juvenile rheumatoid arthritis, sexual activity, and possible problems can be discussed during the initial visit, with the comment that questions are welcome at any time Referral to one of the many peer self-help groups for social interaction may help, if he or she seems isolated. If the patient is older and married, an initial interview with each partner separately, then as a couple, assists evaluation of marital and sexual problems. Questions should be asked about changes in sexual functioning since the arthritis developed and these should be explicit: about the frequency per month of intercourse, preferred positions, masturbation, desire, and morning erections.

Sexual problems may predate the arthritis and represent a longstanding difficulty, requiring referral for sexual counselling and therapy. On the other hand some couples temporarily reduce coital frequency only during an acute phase of arthritis, an adjustment that neither distresses them nor implies dysfunction. Probably the most important suggestions to give to a patient with arthritis, concern comfortable *positions for coitus*. The simple recommendation of placing a pillow under painful limbs can be helpful. The physician can use little pipe cleaner 'dolls' (blue for male, pink for female) to demonstrate possible new positions, and these are much easier to understand than verbal explanation. Both partners should be asked if they understand and if they think they will be able to achieve the suggested position at home. They may even invent their own and tell the doctor who may thus help the next couple.

For example, many couples appreciate learning a non-weight-bearing, partially lateral position, in which both partners recline with trunks at right angles to one another. They face one another legs intertwining, so that breast and genital play is possible. The penis enters the vagina at the '4 p.m.' or '8 p.m.' position, where the pudendal nerve is entering on either side. Another suggestion is for the male arthritic to recline while the non-arthritic female partner straddles him in the superior position. She often needs the physician's encouragement and reassurance, because to women unaccustomed to this position, it may seem too exposed; to a shy insecure man, it may seem too demanding and, therefore, threatening. He may need reassurance and encouragement to relax and enjoy being receptive. A helpful suggestion for the patient with limited movement of the hips is a manoeuvre with the acronym FABER: flexion, abduction, external rotation of the legs. In other words, rather than attempting to separate the extended legs, the person draws the legs up with the knees bent and then spreads the knees apart.

When arthritis is so severe that spreading the legs apart is painful or awkward and the patient has difficulty in moving the wrist or hand, adequate washing of the perineum may be difficult. The physician might then suggest that the healthy partner make genital washing part of the sexual foreplay. This can involve a warm soapy bath and use of a hand shower on the genitals. This measure can also prevent poor hygiene from becoming a negative factor in the couple's sex life.

Basic sex therapy is to suggest plenty of sensual, affectionate, non-genital foreplay, avoiding pressure on painful joints. The use of skin lotion is good for arthritic couples. If the patient is fatigued in the evening and feels this interferes with pleasurable sexual exchange, then it is better to utilize early morning for intercourse. A preliminary shared hot bath can be pleasant, relax the joints while also being fun and quite erotic, with the couple going back to bed after bathing. It is important to remind them that emptying the bladder allows for more comfortable loveplay and sexual exchange. Some arthritic patients who are taking analgesics may prefer to take a dose before loveplay, but others feel that this reduces sensation and so prefer to make love first and take the medication later. Additional jelly lubrication may be suggested if a woman has atropic vaginal changes or diminished mucus secretion because of Sjogren's syndrome, which might be part of her rheumatoid arthritis (Engleman and Silverman 1979). Saliva is also satisfactory for lubrication and perfectly safe, natural, and normal to use, although some may need reassurance about this.

When sexual intercourse is simply not possible by reason of physical disability, it is helpful to explain and discuss the limitations of arthritis, and encourage such sexual alternatives as caressing, cuddling, holding, and being held. A discussion with both partners about mutual masturbation and oral sexual contact helps both and they may be invited to ask questions about these sexual alternatives. They should be encouraged to air their fears about ageing and about loss of mobility and independence; the important thing is to achieve honest and loving communication between the partners. Sharing individual fears can lead to mutual support, affection, and closeness. Referral of a couple to a marital or sex therapist depends on a physicians comfort and interest in providing the sex education outlined here, and the availability in the community of competent sex therapists who understand both the physical limitations of arthritics and the sexual side-effects of their medications. Back-up consultation by the rheumatologist then is essential for couple and counsellor.

INFLUENCE OF ALCOHOL

Alcoholics, often but mistakenly, are thought to be sexually liberated. While moderate social drinking frequently facilitates sex by reducing inhibitions, heavy alcohol consumption results in transient physical effects. Alcohol is not a stimulant. For a brief period it acts as a euphoriant, dissolving caution and inhibitions, and then it acts as a depressant of the autonomic and central nervous systems, causing drowsiness, delayed or partial erections, or delayed ejaculations (Lemere and Smith 1973; Masters and Johnson 1970; Roundtable 1970; Shuckit 1972). In the brain, alcohol is a chemical depressant and can directly inhibit sexual responses. Within the autonomic nervous system, an imbalance of cholinergic and adrenergic nerve fibres can affect the sexual cycle of acutely intoxicated men or women. The peripheral nerves carry mixed autonomic nerve fibres, and peripheral neuropathy as a side-effect of alcohol can cause impotence. In fact, alcohol is the most common cause of the first episode of secondary impotence. Further anxiety about impotence may then continue beyond the drinking experience, and may lead to psychogenic impotence. Therefore, careful questioning while taking a sexual history is important in seeking the problem's origin.

Chronic alcoholism

Chronic alcoholism may be defined as drinking that interferes with one's life, involving personal, legal, physical, and job-related problems. The physician should not overlook a clinical depression, which may be related to the patient's sexual symptoms. Women with chronic alcoholism may have sexual problems, although they rarely volunteer this information to physicians, whom they may visit with other priorities (Shuckit 1972). Women alcoholics not uncommonly become prostitutes to earn money for alcohol. In chronically alcoholic men, sexual dysfunction may range from partial erection to permanent secondary impotence, and may be manifest as non-ejaculation as well as delayed ejaculation. Vascular complications related to concomitant diseases, such as diabetes, hypertension, internal iliac atherosclerosis, may affect sexual functioning, but only if the angiopathy is severe (Hellerstein and Friedman 1970; Renshaw 1979*b,c*).

Hormonal changes may follow if there are liver changes, with resultant lowered testosterone and this may produce libido problems. Cirrhosis may lead to gynaecomastia, testicular atrophy, oligospermia, and loss of body hair. Also, prolactin levels may be raised and sexual dysfunctions may follow, whilst a clinical depression may additionally complicate alcoholism. If reduced libido is caused by depression associated with alcoholism, the sexual drive should return following about 4 weeks without alcohol consumption and with adequate medication — doxepin or amitriptyline (50–200 mg of either drug at bedtime). The single large dose assists sleep, making a hypnotic redundant. Abstinence from alcohol does not eliminate all sexual dysfunctions related to heavy drinking. The reasons why sex problems for some alcoholics are resolved when they are 'dry', while for others they are not, remain unknown. In fact, some 8 per cent of alcoholics begin to experience dysfunction for the first time when they stop drinking (Lemere and Smith 1973). Could this be because of passive retaliation towards the spouse, or return of sexual inhibitions 'drowned' in alcohol? Each case must be evaluated and marital counselling may be of benefit.

PHYSICAL DISORDERS

Cardiac disease

Patients with cardiac disease and hypertension until recently have received little help from physicians regarding their many sexual fears (Hellerstein and Friedman 1970). Many questions, such as the following, reflect their concerns. 'Will I have another coronary attack?' 'Will I have a stroke during intercourse?' 'Will I die?' 'Will I be a failure at sex?'

First of all, the physician needs an in-depth, pre-illness sex history, which includes frequency, preferred positions, intercoital masturbation, morning erections, and so forth. Sexual activity can be influenced by libido, angina, the spouse's health and co-operation, the patient's physical state, alcohol intake and necessary medications (digitalis, diuretics, tranquillizers, and β-blockers). Sexual problems may also result from psychological factors related to anxiety, ageing, depression, anger at the spouse or the self, and deliberate suppression of sexual feelings.

Sexual arousal raises the blood pressure and heart rate about as much as does climbing 20 stairs (Hellerstein and Friedman 1970). The physical activity of intercourse (with one's own familiar partner) uses only about seven calories per minute, totalling 30–185 calories. Anxiety and anger raise blood pressure and heart rate a great deal more than sex does. The majority of reported coital coronaries (80 per cent) occur in an unfamiliar place with an unfamiliar partner (presumably such sex representing an attempt to deny ageing or illness and affirm attractiveness). Fear of discovery, sexual excitement, or anxiety about performing well for a new partner may produce excessive noradrenaline secretion, an important aetiological factor in coronary attacks.

The physician should convey relevant sexual information to patient and spouse and answer their questions truthfully. When the patient can manage to climb two flights of stairs comfortably, coitus is safe. The patient may be told that since masturbation raises the heartbeat and blood pressure a little more than coitus does, a restored (conflict-free) intercourse is advantageous. However, in the absence of a partner, or if there are severe marital problems, masturbation may be the optimum sexual expression for the patient. For the hypertensive patient, the supine position is preferable to standing, since lying down will mean a reduction in blood pressure. Finally, adjustments in medications such as: diuretics, diazepam, dilantin, guanethidine sulfate, methyldopa, or reserpine may be necessary if these are found to be causing potency problems (Masters and Johnson 1970).

Strokes

If cerebrovascular disease leads to a paralytic stroke producing hemiplegia, the physician should take a sex history, preferably with both partners present. Unless the stroke was a very severe one, the physician may reassure both partners that sexual function has been spared and that sex, almost as practiced previously, may be resumed. The patient should be informed about sensory changes, i.e. the absence of normal sensation on the affected side of the body. The partners should tell each other what they feel and prefer during sex play. They should be advised that muscular and joint weaknesses on the patient's affected side may indicate the need for a footboard or hand lever to facilitate sexual activities.

Defects in vision, such as homonymous hemianopia, which accompanies a hemiplegia and is irreversible, may prevent recognition of a person or object in the affected visual field. A change in sleeping position in bed by one partner can compensate for this problem. In addition, there may be speech disorders, and under intense sexual desire, for example, the aphasic patient may utter sexual obscenities. Partners should understand and tolerate such occasional outbursts. Post-stroke patients benefit from sexual response rather than sexual avoidance and this can make all the difference in rehabilitation and improving the quality of life after a stroke.

Diabetes

Old medical textbooks stated that 50 per cent of insulin-dependent men who have had diabetes for more than six years will become impotent. Today experts question this assumption which has been challenged (Renshaw 1979 *b,c*). At Loyola Sex Clinic, 26 out of 27 diabetic patients on insulin for 15–17 years, experienced reversal of secondary impotence of 2–7 years' duration, within 2–7 weeks. There certainly may be minimal orgasmicity in diabetics but there may also be a heavy psychogenic overlay and the latter may be the major factor contributing to secondary impotence, which may, therefore, be reversible. The physician should carefully inquire about morning erections and mastur-bation, as well as about the onset of impotence and the consumption of alcohol.

Endocrine problems have not been found to be related to sexual dysfunction in diabetes, although neuropathy may contribute to sexual problems if marked peripheral neuropathy and dermopathy exist. Sensation of touch and pain should be tested in the pudendal and perianal areas. It is almost impossible to separate neurological and vascular factors in diabetics, since the genital vessels are so closely bound by autonomic nervous control. Angiopathies, usually irreversible, are difficult to study in the penis. Nocturnal penile plethysmog-raphy measures vascular dilation during REM sleep, and may help to differentiate functional from organic impotence, as does penile pulse recording (Renshaw 1979*b,c*). (See also Chapter 5.)

Renal dialysis

In addition to the obvious physical stresses of living in symbiosis with a kidney machine, psychological stresses include fear of disability and death, anxiety about the dependency and possible personal rejection, a sense of isolation, recognition of hostility in others (even murderous impulses in a spouse ambiva-lent about setting up dialysis equipment), and anger about the loss of mobility and control. Multiple social stresses involve loss of various roles; at work, in sports, as a breadwinner, and in sex. The patient's partner, in ignorance, may fear contagion by kiss or coitus. A few follow-up studies show coital frequency to be inversely proportional to the extent of dialysis. Far too little is known about the effects of chronic renal disease on sex, whether the patient's kidney condition is untreated, managed by dialysis or treated by renal transplantation. The physician may assist by educating the patient about kidney disease and its stresses in a realistic manner, whilst the stress produced in both patient and partner can be alleviated by affectionate closeness. The physician should ask explicit questions about their sexual concerns.

Malignant disease

Cancer, tumours, carcinoma, metastasis, malignancy: these are terrifying words to most people, since they conjure up concerns about pain, wasting, weakness, mutilation, dependency, and death. For most there is reality to the distress at a diagnosis of cancer, since few families escape the affliction that the condition brings with it. Some individuals remember, from carrying trays in childhood to a dying grandparent, 'the smell of cancer', which, for example, may have been untreated secondary purulent infection of a corrosive facial cancer.

A woman patient recalled this of her grandfather. She herself at the age of 34 years, developed a panic reaction when she was advised to have a hysterec-tomy due to a grossly abnormal Pap smear 2 weeks previously. Her husband had suddenly developed potency problems in three attempts at intercourse, since she had told him the physician suspected cervical cancer. She became increasingly agitated and anxious, and consciously related this to fear of abandonment by her husband. She was preoccupied with vaginal odours, based not on reality, but on memories of her isolated dying grandfather. She insisted she would rather kill herself than bear her family to suffer nursing of 'me with smelly cancer'. Careful, recurrent, and reassuring medical education, taught her that the subspecialty of oncology has evolved and greatly advanced in the 30 years since her grandfather died. Also that the hysterectomy was preventative only due to a 'pre-malignancy' finding. Later with husband present, they were re-assured that (a) there was no known 'contagion' to the penis, (b) that post-hysterectomy their previously joyous coitus could continue, and (c) further questions were welcome. This allowed them to cope as a couple and, by be-coming supportively closer, handle the crisis.

What if the problem is more serious? Self-concept which closely involves body-image, may be seriously shaken by major surgery. A colostomy, ileostomy, or salivary drooling from facial surgery may cause extra concern about cleanli-ness, secretions, and hygiene. Self-isolation to another bedroom may occur because of shame and in order to avoid rejection by a spouse. The sexually undesirable aspects of excretory bags may be minimized by pre-planning, by a clean towel or towel worn as a cummerband, by humour, and a caring relation-ship, both between the couple themselves, and on the part of a sensitive surgeon and physician, who can do much to assist couples in their difficult task of facing malignancy. Disenfranchizing them sexually may only hamper a healthy restoration of the life we have tried to save.

SURGICAL OPERATIONS

Any surgery 'down there' such as: hernia repair, haemorrhoid removal, hyster-ectomy, varicocoele, or even varicose vein stripping, are all known to have caused anxiety and doubt about sexual potency and desirability, to the point of dysfunction. Prostatectomy surgery is perhaps for men the best known cause of distress, because for about 10–30 per cent of men prostatectomy results in retrograde ejaculation, due to inevitable damage to the internal bladder sphincter. Failure to see and feel the familiar external ejaculate may cause a man to panic, think 'that's it, I'm ruined sexually', and give up with psychogenic impotence without even talking to his urologist surgeon.

Some women (and their partners) believe a myth that 'women become fat and sexless' after hysterectomy, which may unfortunately become, quite need-lessly, a self-fulfilling prophecy if they nervously avoid each other in bed. A sensitive gynaecologist, urologist, or general surgeon must be aware of these possibilities, in order to set aside an extra half hour both *before* and *after* surgery, to ask the same open-ended question: 'Do you have any sexual concerns about the operation?' Explicit dialogue, an illustrative diagram, encouragement, and reassurance yield high therapeutic dividends in return for the valuable time spent on such patient (and partner) sex and body education.

CONCLUSIONS

For men strongly desirous of potency, the last decade has evolved a modern surgical help: inflatable or rigid penile prostheses (Renshaw 1979a). They are expensive and not without risks, both physical and psychological. A fine surgical outcome may disturb a couple's adjustment, if the wife is unwilling and un-receptive of the implanted prosthesis. Thus an adverse interpersonal outcome may result and even lead to divorce. On the other hand, if both are informed of what to expect, the mechanical help may make the husband delighted to be able to feel he is again an effective 'penetrator'. The wife may be pleasured and also pleased that he is pleased. Both, therefore, must be part of the 'before, during, and after' surgery programme to ensure optimal use of the costly device, which some men have inserted but do not later use sexually.

Both husband and wife deserve to know as much as possible about their body's sexual responses to ageing, medications, illnesses, and surgery, together with what sexual therapy, both surgical and non-surgical, may be available. Patients are today *much* less reluctant to discuss their sexual functions than previously presumed by physicians. Emphasizing that 'making sex' can often interfere with 'making love', may go a long way towards guidance of a couple by the physician, to nurturant nearness. Companionship, common interests, and affectionate touching slowly allows them to accept alternatives to coitus, as a joyous way of closeness and intimacy, which greatly reduces the stresses and loneliness they must otherwise face, with ageing, illness, or disability.

References

Busse, E. W. and Pfeiffer, E. (1977). *Behavior and adaptation in late life*. Little, Brown, Boston.

Butler, R. (1975). *Why survive? Being old in America*. Harper & Row, New York.

— — and Lewis, M. (1977). *Sex after sixty*. Harper & Row, New York.

Engleman, E. P. and Silverman, M. (1979). *The arthritis book — a guide for patients and their families*, (Series ed. R. J. Glaser). Painter Hopkins, Sausalito, Ca.

Harman, S. M. and Tsitouras, P. D. (1980). Reproductive hormones in aging men. *J. Clin. Metab. Endocrinol.* **51**, 35–40.

Hellerstein, H. K. and Friedman, E. H. (1970). Sexual activity and the post-coronary patient. *Arch. Int. Med.* **125**, 987–99.

Lemere, F. and Smith, J. W. (1973). Alcohol-induced sexual impotence. *Am. J. Psychiatr.* **130**, 212–13.

Masters, W. and Johnson, V. (1970). *Human sexual inadequacy*. Little, Brown, Boston.

McConnell, A. and Anderson, B. (1978). *Single over 50: how to have the time of your life*, McGraw-Hill, New York.

Renshaw, D. C. (1978). Sex and the senior citizen, *NAPPH J.* **10** (1), 56–61.

— — (1979a). Inflatable penile prosthesis. *JAMA* **241**, 2637–8.

— — (1979b) Diabetic impotence — inevitable or imposed? Part I. *Br. J. Sexual Med.* **6**, 48–51.

— — (1979c). Diabetic impotence — inevitable or imposed? Part II. *Br. J. Sexual Med.* **6**, 35–7.

— — (1981a) Coping with an impotent husband. *Ill. Med. J.* **159**, 29–33.

— — (1981b). A modern view of ancient taboos — masturbation, oral and anal sex. *Consultant* **21** (9), 207–21.

Roundtable (1970). Alcohol, drugs and sex. *MAHS* 18–34, February.

Shuckit, M. A. (1972). Sexual disturbance in the woman alcoholic. *MAHS* 44–65, September.

Tsitouras, P. D. (1982). Relationship of serum testosterone to sexual activity in healthy elderly men. *J. Gerontol.* **37**, 288–93.

Wasow, M. and Loeb, M. B. (1978). Sexuality in nursing homes. In *Sexuality and Aging* (ed. R. L. Solnick) 2nd ed., Ethel Percy Andrus Gerontology Center, Los Angeles, CA.

8
Communication in sex therapy

PATRICIA GILLAN

INTRODUCTION

IF PEOPLE felt able to talk openly about sex there would be far fewer sexual difficulties, since difficulties that are not discussed are frequently not solved. Difficulties that are not solved may cause resentment, which in turn may make communication even more difficult. Of course it is not only sex and sexual feelings that are difficult to talk about, but feelings themselves: feelings of anger and of distress, of suspicion and of love, are all sometimes difficult to discuss openly.

SEX EDUCATION

It is interesting to see how our sexual development takes place and in what context we initially discuss sex. In Europe few schools provide effective sex education and children discuss sex at 'peer level' amongst themselves, usually in a furtive and secretive manner, as though they are discussing something that is dirty or forbidden. C. Farrell (1978) in her book *My Mother Said* pointed out that many such British children are misinformed about sex, as they pass on sexual myths to one another, and that many such children would like to be informed about sex by parents or teachers, but lack this advantage. In Sweden sex education is compulsory from the age of eight, and by nine most Swedish children are sexually well informed compared with English and North American children who, often, at the age of eight, think that a baby emerges from the anus, the navel, or even the mouth. R. and J. Goldman researched children's sexual thinking in their book (Goldman and Goldman 1982), and they concluded that there was a correlation between sex education and knowledge over sexual facts.

Anxieties over sex

Adults find it especially difficult to admit anxiety about a situation which they feel they are expected to face easily. Men, for example, hate to admit anxiety about speaking in public, or about approaching a woman. Women do not like to admit to anxieties concerning their dress or sexual attractiveness. Society lays down standards of competence and adults know what is expected of them in most given circumstances; where they have doubts they often keep quiet out of shame.

In general the rules of sexual conduct are well known; the places where sexual intercourse may take place, for example, are well defined. There are, however, some aspects of sexual behaviour about which many people feel doubtful and therefore anxious, and about which they find it difficult to speak. Oral sex is felt to be wrong or disgusting by some people. Between any couple there are areas where behaviour is not quite certain, and what may seem acceptable to one may be repugnant to the other. These areas need above all to be discussed openly, but unfortunately there still exists a taboo on talking both about feelings and about sex.

The difficulty in talking about feelings extends also to bodies and bodily functions. The Victorians did not like to think of themselves as animals, and in order to affirm their superiority over the animal kingdom, demanded that the animal nature of man be suppressed. Thus it became taboo to expose the body freely, taboo to talk about bodily odours; passing flatus and belching were both extremely bad form, and even the yawn had to be covered. Many of these taboos are being relaxed today: far more of the body may be revealed and there is much more freedom in talking about bodily functions. However, it still remains hard for many people to talk about sex either in public or in private. It is in private that problems arise, and they usually arise where real discussion has not taken place.

The sexual vocabulary

The average person is just not equipped with the technical vocabulary to talk freely about the parts of the body concerned with sex. Learning the vocabulary and learning to overcome the prudery go hand in hand, so that gradually the individual becomes used to or desensitized over a sexual vocabulary. In part the sex therapist begins the treatment by saying, in effect, 'let us learn to talk about sex together'. The therapist who says, 'Do you have oral sex?' is saying firstly that 'oral sex' is a convenient way of referring to oral–genital contact. The act of referring to oral sex represents an encouragement from the therapist to the couple to begin to refer to it in this way.

Gradually, the therapist will proceed to be more specific, and will probably introduce the whole technical vocabulary and demonstrate its use, using various synonyms at the same time. There are occasions when people find it useful to have alternative, more informal expressions, for orgasm and sexual intercourse. The adoption of a casual vocabulary reflected in such expressions as 'to come' and 'to have it', or in basic words such as 'fuck' and 'cunt', probably represents a more relaxed and realistic attitude. Talking about sex in an open way without using formal or vague words inevitably leads to a similar need for frankness in talking about feelings. People often say they do not like doing something, but what exactly do they mean by this? Do they mean that they feel this something to be wrong, or disgusting, or frightening? It is valuable to be able to describe feelings accurately, and to describe them is also, of course, to identify them. In addition, the therapist can also make sure that words describing positive feelings — love, warmth, excitement, etc. — are brought into the talk in a reassuring and approving way. In this way the course of therapy should leave the couple equipped to communicate with ease and facility when talking to one another about emotions and sex.

Regrettably, by the time most people reach adult years the habit of secrecy and reticence over sex is well ingrained. People will often say, 'It just doesn't seem right to talk about it', meaning that they have been thoroughly conditioned not to do so. Unfortunately such an announcement often signifies not only that the subject is closed, but that the mind is too, which means that the problem-solving intellect is denied a chance to change what may be a bad situation. One may also have the problem of one partner being prepared to enter into discussion of sexual matters while the other is not. A woman, for example, has come across some of the newer magazines dealing with sexuality, and wants to start talking about a subject which has not been discussed for years. Her man may immediately feel that he is being criticized in some way, and may react with anger. Or the man, for example, may attempt to open discussion on his wife's 'lack of responsiveness', and she instantly believes that he no longer loves her. If they are unable to get beyond this kind of over-sensitive reaction, a serious barrier to further communication is built up.

Where a therapist becomes involved, time would be spent on reassuring each partner that the expression of suggestions and ideas should not be taken as criticism, but as a means of increasing the pleasure each is able to give and receive.

COMMUNICATION BETWEEN PARTNERS

Often poor sex between partners is caused by a lack of communication over what they both want from each other. In Europe many sex clinics use marital therapy combined with a modified Masters and Johnson (1970, 1979) (M and J) therapy for their out-patients. One of the basic principles of the M and J therapy is that partners learn to communicate non-sexually in the initial stage of their therapy. They are asked to massage one another in a non-sexual manner in the task of 'sensate focusing'. This could be described as non-demanding massage, in which the sexual parts are not touched until the couple have learned to effectively massage each other in non-sexual areas. This is a good opportunity for the couple to learn what they want. The therapist instructs them to give each other feed-back over methods of massage, i.e. if one partner wants to be touched more gently then he or she should tell the other what is required. Positive reinforcement can be given when pleasure is received, and this should be rewarding for the person doing the massage and he or she should learn to 'give to get'. Obviously this type of massage is based on operant conditioning and can be effective, providing a good opportunity to determine how some couples react to each other, especially if they return to the clinic reporting failure. The therapist can then analyse what went wrong and teach the couple to be more observant and sensitive to feed-back from one another.

Genital sensate focusing

Genital sensate focusing is the next stage of sexual communication in the M and J therapy, and here the couple learn to touch each other genitally. One stage that M and J leave out of their treatment package is that of self-focusing, whilst in Europe self-exploration or self-discovery is encouraged, and individuals are given instruction on how to masturbate. Some English women do not know about the location of the clitoris and need to learn where to look for it by the use of diagrams. Such women go through the next stage of how to touch their labia minora and clitoris, and how to find the glans clitoridis. Obviously this stage of self exploration is necessary before partners can communicate what they enjoy. When the woman has discovered her own clitoris she can tell her partner where it is and how she likes to be touched there.

The penis is more obvious to find and touch and perhaps this explains the Masters and Johnson finding, in their book about gay men *Homosexuality in Perspective*, that gay men usually report more effective foreplay than heterosexual couples. This is maybe because men have more experience over masturbating early on. Of course the therapy that is being discussed could be for either a homosexual or a heterosexual couple. We have seen quite a lot of homosexual couples in London and they usually have an underlying 'marital problem' when they undergo sex therapy.

Another stage of GSF (Genital Sensate Focusing) is to tease and prolong genital pleasure by stopping touching and then frustrate the partner before returning to touching the genitals. Obviously this stage needs good communication and co-operation from both partners.

The oral sex stage

Another stage in sex therapy where good communication is called for is the 'oral sex stage'. Many people find the idea of oral sex repugnant. Not only are they ignorant of it, but also shy to experiment with it. The therapist must open the subject with some care and move on from it if resistance is too great. The couple can be reassured on various points. To begin with it is a widespread practice for both sexes, and those who do it are in no way depraved or indeed different from other people. Oral sex has been practised from ancient times and Vatsayana in *The Kama Sutra* refers approvingly to the pleasure of oral sex.

Some people are worried about oral sex being dirty or unhygienic and it is a good idea to get couples to communicate over this aspect. This idea is usually only a rationalization of a deeper repugnance, and it can be pointed out that the mouth itself is in this way similar to the genital regions; both areas normally have many bacteria and other organisms living in them but these organisms do no harm as the healthy body has adequate defences against them. If the couple have never had oral sex, it is a good idea to suggest that they wash first, since this will diminish the strong genital tastes which they may find unpleasant. When a couple are used to oral contact and enjoy it, washing immediately before is unnecessary, providing they wash regularly in any case. It makes no sense to wash away odours which are sexually exciting.

For women who have doubts about oral sex there is the added anxiety that the man may ejaculate into her mouth, and indeed, some women dislike the taste of semen. For a woman who dislikes this there are ways of managing, but communication needs to be effective. She can ask her man to withdraw when orgasm is imminent or judge herself when she should do so. Men who feel ashamed or diffident about ejaculating during fellatio can withdraw a bit early and allow the remainder of the stimulation to be manual.

Women sometimes have the fear that the penile glans will not fit into their mouths or that when it is inside it will press into their throat causing gagging. The woman should be in a position to withdraw the penis the moment deep penetration is threatened. Many women associate fellatio with 'sword swallowing', having seen Linda Lovelace's amazing performance in the film *Deep Throat*. Cunnilingus does not seem to produce so many problems, although some men say they do not like the taste of licking a woman's clitoris. Strong repugnance to oral sex can be overcome by a somewhat frivolous ploy; jam, jelly, or honey is spread on each genital area and each partner takes it in turns to lick it off. It is but a small step to continue licking. There are also some fruit-flavoured lotions available.

Physical examination

It is a good idea to see how partners communicate anxiety or fear when they touch one another, in the context of a two-way physical examination. This can be used as a communication and education exercise, since many people have never examined the genitalia of the opposite sex in real detail. The physical examination will ensure that the therapist and the patients are all talking about the same 'named' parts.

Initially the examination is done by the therapist wearing rubber gloves and then one partner is examined by the other, who need not wear rubber gloves. The examination by the therapist should be leisurely, calm and complete, thus constituting a 'model' for the partner, who then repeats it. To some extent the conduct of the examination is intended as a desensitization for those who may be afraid of touching their partner's or even their own genitals. While each partner is examining the genitals of the other, communication between them may be observed. How do they approach the task? Delicately, roughly, or with about the appropriate touch? Are they nervous or embarrassed? Watch also to see if the patient flinches or draws away, as do women with vaginismus. Both partners are asked to identify each other's genitals and which areas they think are arousing in one another. This task identifies poor communication if one partner mistakenly thinks a certain area is arousing and this is not confirmed by the partner.

Later stages of intercourse

The later stages of sexual intercourse, once all the previous stages have been reached, is another area where communication is crucial. When the therapist discusses the first recommended position of the woman on top, in contrast to the usual missionary position the couple have been using, there is often some hostility on the man's part. He might say that he does not want this position as it might be uncomfortable, when his real fear is that he is going to be dominated by the female. She might find this position unfeminine, as she has been taught that women should be passive when they have sex and should keep still. Maybe she is shocked by the therapist suggesting that she should be

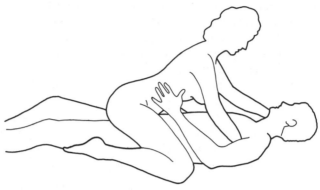

FIG. 8.1 The 'Woman Above' position

active, and when her partner's penis seems to be stiff enough, to guide it into her vagina and move and enjoy the sensations she experiences.

The next position in the M and J repertoire is the 'lateral position', but in the UK we have found that many patients find this difficult to manage. Initially we thought this might be due to poor communication, but as a result of personal experiences, problems certainly do arise. Accordingly, we recommended the 'Feel Free Position' with which people experience no difficulties. The 'Feel Free Position' is an important position for the therapy of orgasmic dysfunction, as the woman is free to enjoy some manual stimulation of the clitoris, provided by herself or her partner. This position is associated with good communication between both partners and leads to pleasure.

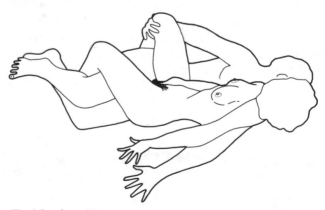

FIG. 8.2 The 'Feel free' position

Various techniques for certain sexual problems rely on good communication. The Squeeze technique and the Stop-Start technique for premature ejaculation rely on good communication, as the partners should give feedback to each other, especially where one partner needs to keep still to learn ejaculatory control and the other partner needs to accept this and fully co-operate. It is quite easy for an unco-operative partner to sabotage a sex therapy programme, for example putting the teasing technique into practice during sensate focusing, where stimulation is stopped for a while and then recommenced. Poor communication can lead to doing this too late, etc. In anorgasmia good communication leads to both partners being fully aware of arousal and the state of affairs between them, in relation to the provided stimulation being suitable and effective.

Contract therapy

Bad communication between partners can lead to disappointing sex and poor non-sexual relations as well. The possibilities of poor interaction between two people are endless and range from minor irritations, proceeding by all stages to violence or mental cruelty. Relationships can become very complex; partners may have taken up positions of no retreat, and it is only too easy to get hopelessly involved or confused.

Communication difficulties are approached in two ways. In the first, patients are encouraged to improve their sexual interaction and communication, and the relationship will improve as a consequence. This is very often true. The other approach is to consider carefully the area of concern and see if some simple analysis may suggest a 'give to get' solution. At a very simple level, where both partners have, shall we say, a niggling complaint about the other, an exchange agreement can be negotiated. For example: 'If you will tell me the details of the family finances so that I can play a part in them, I will be more willing to help entertain your friends'; or perhaps at a deeper level: 'If you spend some time talking with me, I will try to put some enthusiasm into my sex life'; or again: 'I will come out with you more often if you will show more interest in the children'. Any couple may have numerous areas of disagreement which may be paired off in this way.

When this approach is made systematic it is called 'Contract Therapy'. The couple are remotivated to make certain sacrifices in the interests of greater harmony and sexual co-operation. But it must be presented positively so that the tasks are requested and not forbidden (*not* 'I won't sleep with you unless . . .').

Communication therapy

It may also be a valuable lesson to teach a couple how to talk to one another. Previous discussions may have failed because the couple could not keep up a dialogue without quarrelling. This may be because one partner, or both, begin to feel threatened in some way and retreat into sulking, hostility, or pretended indifference. The therapist may suggest ways of overcoming this. One method is to set aside a time each week for communication therapy when it is a rule to keep calm. Another rule could be to break off the discussion at a given time, and not to try to solve everything at one go. Another good method used in marital therapy is to get each partner to listen to the other and to repeat what the partner has said, to test that communication has actually taken place.

This method of communication training is useful and effective. Crowe, Gillan, and Golombok (1981) carried out a Maudsley study in which Masters and Johnson type therapy (modified) was compared with marital/communication therapy. Forty eight couples with impotence, anorgasmia, or loss of libido were randomly allocated to one of three treatment conditions:

(i)   modified M and J with a male and a female therapist.

(ii) modified M and J with only one therapist.

(iii) marital/communication therapy and relaxation comparison procedure with one therapist.

The major variables investigated were type of therapy (comparing M and J with marital/communication therapy), number of therapists (one or two), and sex of therapist. Post-treatment and one year follow up assessments showed no significant difference in outcome between treatment approaches. No significant effects were found for sex of therapist, or for the interaction between sex of therapist and sex of presenter. Marital contracts were of the 'give and get' variety (Crowe 1978).

SOCIAL SKILLS TRAINING

Many more people who do not have partners are presenting themselves at sex therapy clinics requesting help. Often they do not have partners because they have lacked the necessary skill to acquire a partner, and want to know how to change their state of non-interaction and social isolation. Many people lack the ability to communicate and thereby to control important events in their daily lives. For example, people who communicate badly often talk in a rather quiet voice and find it difficult to look directly into the eyes of the person to whom they are talking. They may also find it difficult to express their emotions openly and this applies equally to love and to anger. This is often related to a lack of assertion.

In a marital partnership an inability to be a good communicator may have serious results. The poor communicating partner may feel a helpless resentment, which may easily amount to a passive hostility manifesting itself as a lack of warmth, a lack of enthusiasm, a lack of sexual co-operation and initiative, or perhaps as sulking or moodiness.

Assertion training

Methods have been developed in the last decade to deal with this problem and are generally referred to as assertion training or personal effectiveness therapy (Argyle 1969; Liberman *et al.* 1975). These techniques may be administered by a single therapist, but they are usually taught in a group situation, that is with therapists and a group of patients. The training is based on advice and practice, the therapist giving direct advice on how to behave, and then demonstrating what has been suggested. The therapist might, for example, say to the patient: 'When you are talking with your wife you should adopt a patient but firm attitude; you must try to look her straight in the eye from time to time. Watch while I show you how to do this and then you have a try'. This demonstration of behaviour is called modelling. If the wife is complaining of her husband's overbearing manner, the female therapist can take the role of the wife and maintain a more assertive attitude in a mock argument with the real husband. When the 'model' of assertion has been demonstrated, the wife may try it herself in the presence of the therapists. Similarly, if the husband complains that he finds it difficult to show affection, the male therapist can give a demonstration by putting his arm around the female therapist in an appropriately warm manner, together with other suitable expressions. Then this 'model' may be enacted by the man with his partner. Suggestions and discussion can always follow.

The accent is always kept on encouragement and reward and not upon criticism. Even when a patient clearly fails in some way, the therapist should only remark: 'I am sure you will do better next time', or perhaps draw attention to some way in which the patient did succeed, however small, such as: 'You smiled nicely that time'.

The lone individual

Often it is more difficult to teach communication training to individuals who have never had a partner or even a friend. Liberman *et al.* (1975) has researched methods for dealing with such people and he calls his method 'Personal Effectiveness training', as opposed to assertion or aggression training, since the aim of the therapy is to enable people to mix with and communicate effectively with other people. The therapist initially can set up a staged enactment of such a situation in front of the group and members of the group can model this later. The group task could be to enter a room where a party is to be held, and find a stranger to converse with. Role rehearsal is for each member of the group to team up with another member and talk with another group member, changing every 5 min to another person.

Another more advanced task is for the therapists to demonstrate how to 'make a date'. Then the most confident group member can try the 'date' task and model his or her behaviour on the therapist, in front of the group. The therapist always finds some praise of the attempt, even though it might have been a far from perfect performance. For example: 'You could look at her more' or: 'Smile more'. Each member of the group gets a turn to act out his or her difficulty, re-enacting the same scene until his performance improves and he gains confidence. Further tasks may consist of dating and sexual skills, all based on 'role rehearsal' and modelling methods. We have carried out some social skills/communication work at Guys Hospital and, together with Yaffe (Gillan and Yaffe 1981), agree with Sol Gordon (1979) over two essential ingredients in interactions; having a sense of humour and taking an interest in a subject other than oneself. We have found that 9 out of 10 men who were given role rehearsal and systematic desensitization therapy, made progress in dating and had a clearly more hopeful attitude towards their sexuality (Gillan 1976). Some visited massage parlours to get used to physical contact, to put their relaxation into practice, to enjoy being touched, and to communicate to the masseuse their preferences with regard to the sites of massage. Others benefited by joining an Encounter Group.

A group of single people without partners was researched at Guys Hospital by Gillan and Yaffe (1981). Seven out of eight of the people in the group suffered from psychological disabilities: mainly social and sexual phobias. Group therapy methods consisted of relaxation techniques, sharing and discussing problems, rehearsing situations in which people meet, assertion training, role playing, social skills and homework tasks. The two therapists rehearsed social situations in which the patients' tasks were carefully graded, so that each week group members could gain confidence until they could 'make a date'. Later sexual behaviour was described with the help of slides. Results for this group of one woman and seven men showed that an improvement in 6 out of 8 patients took place 4 months after therapy. This improvement was associated with attendance at social events and the finding of suitable contacts. This finding was not apparent at the end of therapy; it seems that a 'consolidation period' is necessary for patients to benefit.

GROUP THERAPY AND COMMUNICATION

Group sex therapy techniques became an established form of therapy in the UK in the late 1970s on the National Health Service. Women's group therapy (Gillan, Golombok, and Becker 1980) is well established and is based on sex education and communication techniques. The woman who has situational anorgasmia with her partner but is orgasmic when she masturbates alone, can learn to communicate her desires to her partner. Role playing can be helpful in the women's group, or each woman can be given homework to practise in the telling of what she wants to her husband or partner. Furthermore, she can practise doing this in front of a mirror before actually rehearsing this in the group and later with her partner at home. Group feedback is useful in this type of case and the women can help each other to communicate more effectively. Many women are taught to be passive in their culture and often they do nothing about initiating sex when they feel like it, waiting for their partner to suggest it. Obviously this is an example of poor communication, and role playing can help such a woman to learn to take the initiative. Other women are embarrassed about asking their partners to say certain things or carry out certain acts during foreplay, and again role playing and discussion in the group can help. Yet again, other women are afraid of saying 'no' when the partner suggests making love. Once again role playing of saying 'no' in the group, can be helpful.

Male sex therapy

Men's sex therapy groups have been organized by Gillan and Yaffe (1981) along the lines advocated by Zilbergeld (1979), and since 1977 about 24 men with erectile and/or ejaculatory problems have attended such groups. Several men with sex problems were severely handicapped by their lack of social and communication skills, and needed to be helped initially in a social skills group before graduating to a men's sex therapy group. Results are shown in Table 8.1.

Therapy consists of imagery and body control and the men are given homework along Zilbergeld's lines, during which they practice fantasy shaping, relaxation, and body control, and also learn to enjoy their sensations. Part of the therapy is related to communication training. Most men do not communicate

TABLE 8.1 *Results of group sex therapy in British men*

Problem	Much improved	Improved	Same	Worse	Total
Secondary erectile dysfunction (SED)		1	1	1	3
SED + premature ejaculation	1	4			5
Premature ejaculation		4	2		6
Retarded ejaculation	1	1			2
Inexperienced	1		2		3
Total	3	10	5	1	19

68% improved

about sex honestly with one another, and consequently various sexual myths are spread about male sexuality; a similar manifestation to 'machismo'.

We discuss male sexual myths and concentrate on Zilbergeld's list:

Myth 1: Men should not have, or at least not express certain feelings.

Myth 2: In sex, as elsewhere, it is performance that counts.

Myth 3: The man must take charge of an orchestrate sex.

Myth 4: A man always wants and is always ready to have sex.

Myth 5: All physical contacts must lead to sex.

Myth 6: Sex equals intercourse.

Myth 7: Sex requires an erection.

Myth 8: Good sex is a linear progression of increasing excitement terminated only by orgasm.

Myth 9: Sex should be natural and spontaneous.

Myth 10: In this enlightened age, the preceding myths no longer have any influence on us.

The men are asked to discuss these myths in the group and are often quite surprised how well they can be applied to a British culture. Some of Zilbergeld's exercises are based on social skills training and the men roleplay saying 'no' to a non-sexual request from a partner, or saying 'no' to a sexual request.

CONCLUSIONS

Behaviour modification methods are effective when applied to problems of communication between people, couples with sexual difficulties and relationship problems. Such therapy can be given individually, conjointly or in a group situation and one of the most important variables is that of role playing, whilst modelling is also useful. More research needs to be carried out to improve communication skills in people, and it is apparent that video tape methods will have a useful part to play in achieving this end.

References

Argyle, M. (1969). *Social interaction*. Methuen, London.

Crowe, M. J. (1978). Conjoint marital therapy: a controlled outcome study. *Psychol. Med.* **8**, 623–36.

—— Gillan, P. and Golombok, S. (1981). Form and Content in the conjoint treatment of sexual dysfunction: a controlled study. *Behav. Res. Ther.* **19**, 47–54.

Farrell, C. (1978). *My mother said . . . : the way young people learned about sex and birth control.* Routledge & Kegan Paul, London.

Gillan, P. and Gillan, R. (1976). *Sex therapy today.* Open Books, London.

–– Golombok, S., and Becker, P. (1980). NHS sex therapy groups for women. *Br. J. Sex. Med.* 7, 44–7.

–– and Yaffe, M. (1981). Group therapy for men. *Br. J. Sex. Med.* 8, 35–7.

Goldman, R. and Goldman, J. (1982). *Children's sexual thinking.* Routledge & Kegan Paul, London.

Gordon, S. (1979). *The New You.* Bantam Books, London.

Liberman, R. P. (1975). *Personal Effectiveness.* Research Press, New York.

Masters, W. H. and Johnson, V. E. (1970). *Human sexual inadequacy.* Livingstone, Edinburgh.

–– –– (1979). *Homosexuality in perspective.* Little, Brown, Boston.

Zilbergeld, B. (1979). *Men and sex.* Little, Brown, Boston.

9

Sexual dysfunction in alcoholic men

I. KARACAN AND C. A. MOORE

INTRODUCTION

CHRONIC ALCOHOLICS and intoxicated non-alcoholics frequently report changes in sexual desire, erectile capabilities, and ejaculatory function. The alterations in these three areas of sexuality are dependent on blood alcohol concentration (BAC), duration, pattern, and extent of drinking, and a number of other factors, such as premorbid sexual functioning, age, and attendant psychopathology or medical illness. A major difficulty in comparing the available studies is the lack of this information about the patient population and control subjects. The wide inter- and intra-individual variation of drinking patterns makes research quantification of alcohol consumption, an obviously important variable in the study of alcohol-related impotence, quite difficult. Chronic alcohol consumption is not a variable that can be controlled in human studies, and there is no adequate animal model for studying penile erectile capability. Further complicating interpretation of the data are differences in methodology, and at times, even a lack of definition of which aspect of sexuality is being considered, e.g. libido, erection, or ejaculation. The focus of this chapter is alcohol-related erectile failure: impotence.

ALCOHOL AND PENILE ERECTION

Several studies have relied on survey or questionnaire data to study the effects of alcohol on penile erections. Lemere and Smith (1973) state that 'at least eight percent' of alcoholic male inpatients complained of impotence. However, it is unclear whether they specifically asked patients in a systematic way, and if so, how many male patients were questioned. A much higher percentage of patients will endorse having had 'difficulty in obtaining or maintaining erections' than will acknowledge 'impotence'; so the phrasing of the question affects the results of the survey. For example, Whalley (1973) reports that 54 per cent of 50 hospitalized male alcoholics and 28 per cent of healthy controls complained of having had erectile failure at some time. Still another survey of hospitalized male alcoholics (Powell, Viamontes, and Brown 1974) reports that 4 per cent of alcoholics and no controls complained of 'erectile problems' while sober and 24 and 10 per cent, respectively, had such problems while intoxicated. Akhtar (1977) reports a 31 per cent prevalence of impotence in a group of alcoholics who were admitted to a detoxification unit.

As the previous paragraph illustrates, survey and interview data can vary markedly from one study to another. A more objective approach to quantifying alcohol-related erectile function is through laboratory evaluation. Gantt (1940, 1952) and Teitelbaum and Gantt (1958) observed erections in dogs obtained by penile manipulation after a variety of doses of alcohol. They found that ability both to obtain and maintain erections decreased with increasing dose of ethanol. As mentioned earlier, however, animal penile tumescence studies cannot be assumed to be applicable to human function, because of important anatomical, physiological, and psychological differences.

Several studies of the effects of ethanol on erectile function in humans have used fantasy and erotic films, and measured erections with a penile strain gauge. Rubin and Henson (1976) gave placebo and ethanol beverages to 16 healthy male subjects, finding that mean size of erections was significantly reduced at ethanol doses of 0.5, 1.0, and 1.5 ml/kg of 100 proof vodka. Peak erection size was reduced and latency to erection increased significantly only at the 1.5 ml/kg dose. Farkas and Rosen (1976) and Bridell and Wilson (1976) also found a negative linear relationship between penile tumescence and alcohol consumption in healthy subjects during an erotic film. The former authors noted that there was some increase in maximal penile diameter at a low BAC (0.025 per cent), possibly due to decreased inhibition in the laboratory setting.

There is little objective information about erectile function in chronic alcoholics. A study undertaken by ourselves addresses itself to the effects of chronic alcoholism on the nocturnal penile tumescence (NPT) of sober alcoholics. The method of NPT monitoring and its advantages over other means of evaluation of erectile capacity are described in Chapter 5. The data presented here have been presented in part previously (Snyder and Karacan 1981).

An experimental investigation

Patients admitted to the Houston VA Medical Center gave informed written consent for participation in the study and were initially placed in the alcohol detoxification unit. Three weeks after detoxification was complete (i.e. patients were receiving no psychotropic medications and were physically stable) evaluation for inclusion in the study was conducted. Patients underwent a complete history and physical evaluation and an extensive battery of laboratory tests including electrocardiography (ECG), urinalysis, complete blood count (CBC), blood chemistries (SMA 20), and serology. Patients were specifically excluded if they manifested organic brain syndrome, major or minor depressive disorder, schizophrenia, or other thought disorder. None of the subjects or controls met the criteria for inhibited sexual desire, inhibited sexual excitement, or inhibited male orgasm as defined by DSM-III (1980) and secured through a standardized sexual history (GAP Report No. 88, 1973). Known cardiac, hepatic, renal, and endocrine diseases were not present and all liver function tests were normal throughout the course of the study. The patients received no medications during the investigation.

Patients were included if they were between 25 and 55, demonstrated major alcoholism as defined by the National Council on Alcoholism (1972) and were devoid of a primary sleep disorder (i.e. narcolepsy, sleep apnoea, etc.). The mean number of years of alcoholism was 7.2, with a range of 3-15 years. On admission to the hospital, 22 (85 per cent) patients exhibited physiological dependence (definite withdrawal symptoms of hallucinations, clouded sensorium, withdrawal seizures, autonomic hyperactivity and/or severe tremulousness). Eight (30 per cent) drank despite previous medical contraindications, 23 (88 per cent) drank despite clear social contraindications (i.e. job loss, arrest for intoxication), and 24 (92 per cent) had a history of tolerance to alcohol. The percentage of patients with two of these criteria was 82 per cent and with three or more, 63 per cent. These factors comprise diagnostic level one of the National Council on Alcoholism criteria and are associated with alcoholism in a 'clear, definite, classical, and obligatory way'.

Diagnositc level two of the criteria is indicative of probable frequent alcohol abuse and is characteristic of chronic alcoholism. The number and percentage of patients with these criteria were as follows: alcoholic blackout periods (14, 54 per cent), complaint of loss of control of alcohol consumption (18, 69 per cent), vascular engorgement of the face (12, 46 per cent), surreptitious drinking (19, 73 per cent), morning drinking (16, 62 per cent), spouse complaining about drinking (11 of 15, 73 per cent), repeated attempts at abstinence (17, 65 per cent), changing from one alcoholic beverage to another (14, 54 per cent), and outbursts of rage and suicidal ideation while drinking (62 per cent).

A total of 287 patients were screened for inclusion. Of these, 77 were excluded for psychological reasons and 176 for physical reasons, whilst 14 were excluded for both. Thirty met the standards for inclusion. However, two patients left the hospital prior to completing the study, one patient developed an upper respiratory infection, and one patient was diagnosed by polysomnographic evaluation as having sleep apnoea. These four were excluded, giving a final sample of 26, representing 9 per cent of the patients originally screened. Each patient was matched by age (± 3 years) with a healthy control subject who had undergone similar NPT monitoring. Controls could have a history of mild social drinking only.

Parameters of penile change

Changes in penile circumference were determined by mercury-filled strain gauges (Karacan 1969) that were attached to the penis. One gauge was placed around the tip just below the glans and one at the base of the penis. Changes in penile circumference were directly reflected on the polygraph tracing by deflections from baseline.

Tumescence tracings were scored according to the following rules: a tumescence episode is judged to be present when a deviation on the tumescence tracing attains an amplitude of at least 20 per cent of the greatest amplitude recorded for the particular subject and lasts at least 20 s. Each tumescence episode is classified as either a maximum or semi episode. For a maximum episode, the circumference of the penis is between 81 and 100 per cent of the greatest circumference recorded for the subject. For a semi episode, the circumference is between 20 and 80 per cent of the greatest circumference recorded for the subject. Additionally, the erection judged to be the greatest was measured for rigidity. If the penis buckled at pressures less than 450 g, the tumescence was considered a semi episode and no episodes were termed maximum, regardless of circumference change. During an episode the penis may attain maximum tumescence for a while, become flaccid, then reattain some degree of tumescence. Such events are classified according to the length of the transient period of flaccidity and the degree of tumescence reattained during this period. If the penis becomes flaccid for 1 min or longer, the event is classified as two distinct episodes.

Alcoholic subjects were evaluated on two consecutive nights. On the second night, subjects were awakened during the first maximal tumescence episode, the penis was photographed and buckling pressure measured by means of a specially designed pressure device. A penis of sufficient rigidity to ensure penetration will not buckle with pressures less than 450 g.

All-night sleep electroencephalogram (EEG) and electro-oculogram (EOG) were monitored on the study nights and subjects did not nap during the day. A standard bipolar half-montage electrode placement (F1–F7; P1–T5; O3–OzPz; left eye to nasion; nasion to right eye) was used, and scored according to the method of Williams, Agnew, and Webb (1964). EEG–EOG tracings were scored blindly with respect to patient and study condition and each 1-min epoch of an EEG–EOG tracing was scored as 1 of 6 stage categories: sleep stages 1, 2, 3, 4, REM, or the waking stage. Values for 21 standard sleep parameters were then generated from these data (Williams, Karacan, and Hursch, 1974).

Results of the study

Data from the two groups were compared with two-tailed t-tests for independent samples. A probability (P) of 0.05 was the limit for statistical significance.

TABLE 9.1 *Parameters of nocturnal penile tumescence (NPT)*

	Patients (n = 26)		Controls (n = 26)		P <
Age	40.0	7.9	40.0	8.7	NS
Total tumescence time (min)	110.5	57.9	118.0	46.9	NS
Tumescence latency (min)	96.7	56.9	145.3	68.8	0.01
Number of maximum erections	1.7	1.4	2.7	1.3	0.02
Amount maximum erections (min)	55.7	50.7	98.2	52.0	0.01
Number of semi-erections	2.5	1.4	1.0	0.7	0.001
Amount semi-erections (min)	54.8	40.7	19.8	15.9	0.001
Simultaneous REM-tumescence (min)	63.9	32.8	69.6	28.9	NS
Maximum circumference (cm)	1.6	0.7	1.9	0.5	NS

Tumescence was clearly impaired in alcoholics as compared to controls, in terms of onset of tumescence and frequency and duration of maximum erections. On average, the beginning of the first tumescence episode occurred about 50 min earlier in the sleep cycles of the patients, as compared to the controls (P < 0.01). There was no significant difference in REM latency between the two groups or in simultaneous REM-tumescence, which is a measure of the amount of tumescence that occurred during REM sleep. Total tumescence time (maximum plus semi) was not significantly different in the two groups. However, the alcoholics had 36 per cent fewer maximum erections and the total duration of these was 43 per cent less than those of controls. The patient group had about 2.5 times the number of partial erections and 2.8 times the duration of these partial erections. This phenomenon of fewer maximum and more partial erections is one we have seen in a variety of patients with organically impaired erectile function.

The sleep of our alcoholic samples was also disturbed in comparison to controls. They spent less time in bed, less time asleep, took more time to fall asleep, and were awake for longer periods of time during the night. However, there were no significant differences in the percentages of the various sleep stages (1, 2, 3, 4, REM). REM sleep was disturbed only in terms of the total number of REM periods during the night, with patients having about one less REM period than controls. This difference may be explained by the significantly decreased total sleep time, since the 84 min less sleep of the alcoholics is somewhat more than the REM interval time. Thus, had the patients slept as long as

TABLE 9.2 *Sleep parameters*

| | Patients | | Controls | | |
	Mean	SD	Mean	SD	P <
Time in bed (min)*	365.9	47.5	428.9	38.2	0.001
Sleep period time (min)†	343.8	47.2	418.5	36.5	0.001
Total sleep time (min)‡	322.3	45.3	405.8	42.5	0.001
Sleep efficiency index (%) §	88.3	7.6	94.6	5.2	0.001
Sleep onset latency (min)	26.7	29.8	8.6	5.9	0.01
Number of awakenings	6.0	4.8	4.5	2.5	NS
REM period length (min)	28.1	9.1	25.0	6.1	NS
REM interval length (min)	67.3	14.0	63.0	12.1	NS
Number of REM periods	3.5	1.0	4.5	0.9	0.001
% Stage 0	6.1	6.2	3.1	4.2	0.05
% Stage 1	4.7	2.5	6.2	3.3	(0.10)
% Stage 2	50.5	9.2	54.8	8.7	(0.10)
% Stage 3	4.8	4.0	5.4	3.3	NS
% Stage 4	6.5	8.0	4.7	5.7	NS
% Stage REM	27.4	6.9	25.8	6.4	NS
Latency to first awakening (min)	86.7	116.4	165.9	132.6	0.05
Latency to stage REM (min)¶	67.1	37.5	77.4	27.5	NS
Latency to stage 2 (min)	9.7	13.9	7.4	6.2	NS
Latency to stage 3 (min)	44.6	35.9	32.4	23.1	NS
	(n = 21)‖		(n = 23)‖		
Latency to stage 4 (min)	67.1	50.9	35.9	23.8	0.05
	(n = 16)‖		(n = 15)‖		
Latency to arising (min)	1.2	2.5	1.8	3.6	NS

* Time from 'lights out' to arising.
† Time from first entering sleep to last awakening in the morning.
‡ Sleep period time minus duration of night time awakenings.
§ Total sleep time − time in bed.
¶ Latencies to the various stages are measured from sleep onset time.
‖ The number of controls and patients are less than 26 because only the number noted actually had stages 3 and/or 4 sleep.

the controls, the number of REM periods may have been the same. Despite the one less REM period, the REM period length, interval between REM periods and percentage of total sleep time spent in REM sleep, were not notably different in the the two groups. This suggests that REM sleep remained intact in our patients. The patient group had significantly longer latency to stage 4 sleep and we might have expected to see decreased percentages of stages 3 and 4 in the patient group. Our failure to find decreased slow wave sleep (SWS) may be explained by the mean age of patients and controls; at age 40, there is less SWS in the normal population. Also, our patient sample was highly selected for psychological and biological health, relative to the majority of the alcoholics treated on the detoxification unit.

Possible mechanisms of alcohol-related impotence

Possible mechanisms of ethanol related sexual dysfunction have been the focus of much study and even more speculation. Psychological, endocrinological, and neurological dysfunction are most probably involved. A number of studies have evaluated the effect of ethanol on the latter two. Little information exists concerning ethanol-associated psychogenic impotence, probably because of methodological considerations and lack of an animal model. According to Masters and Johnson (1970), 'the second most frequent factor in the onset of secondary impotence can be directly related to a specific incident of acute ingestion of alcohol or to a pattern of excessive alcohol intake *per se*'. These authors suggest that the anxiety generated by a failure of erection during intoxication can lead to continuing psychogenic impotence.

ALCOHOL AND ENDOCRINE FUNCTION

Ethanol in acute and chronic doses can reduce serum testosterone (T) levels in animals and man (Badr and Bartke 1974; Cicero and Badger 1977*a*; Cicero, Meyer, and Bell 1979; Gordon and Southren 1977). There is general agreement in the literature that T levels are decreased in chronic alcoholics with clinical testicular atrophy or hypogonadism. At least four mechanisms may be involved. In chronic alcohol use, degradation of T is enhanced due to induction of hepatic enzymes, in particular, 5-α-reductases. Acute and chronic alcohol use can depress pituitary luteinizing hormone (LH) release, the stimulus for testicular steroidogenesis (Chapin, Breese, and Mueller 1980; Cicero and Badger 1977*b*; Cicero *et al.* 1979; Gordon, Southren, and Lieber 1978; Van Thiel, Lester, and Vaitukaitis 1978), an effect which has not been found in all studies (Wright, Merry, Fry, and Marks 1976; Ylikahri, Huttanen, Harkonen, Leino, Helenius, Liewendahl, and Karonen 1978). A third mechanism may be increased plasma clearance, possibly resulting from reduced plasma protein binding capacity (Gordon, Altman, Southren, Rubin, and Lieber 1976). And finally, ethanol directly inhibits T synthesis despite normal or high LH levels (Cicero *et al.* 1979; Mendelson, Mello, and Ellingboe 1977) although tolerance to this effect may develop. There may also be other mechanisms for decreased T or T-responsiveness in chronic alcoholics, such as disruption of receptor function.

Despite the findings that many alcoholics, particularly those with hypogonadism, have decreased T, many complaining of impotence do not. Thus other mechanisms for sexual dysfunction must be operative.

Prolactin and oestrogen

Alcoholics with gynaecomastia and cirrhosis have elevated prolactin and oestrone levels (Van Theil, Gavaler, Lester, Loriaux and Braunstein, 1975). Basal prolactin levels in non-cirrhotic alcoholics are low, but show exaggerated responses to thyrotropin-releasing hormone, a releasing agent for prolactin. Elevated prolactin and oestrogen levels are associated with decreased libido, and hyperprolactinaemia has been associated with impotence (Cunningham, Karacan, Ware, Lantz and Thornby 1982; Avman and Karacan unpublished data). However, alcoholics with cirrhosis and gynaecomastia were excluded from our study.

Neural dysfunction

Integrity of the nervous system, central and peripheral, is necessary for normal penile erections. The central 'centres' for erection in humans are not known, but cortical and subcortical areas are involved. Lesioning of the frontal cortex, temporal lobes, limbic system, septal area, thalamus, and hypothalamus, and certain brainstem and spinal cord areas, leads to sexual dysfunction. Chronic alcoholics can have damage and neuronal loss in a number of areas of the central nervous system (CNS), such as cortical atrophy, temporal lobe and limbic system damage, and others. However, a causal relationship between alcohol induced CNS damage and erectile failure, if any, has not been demonstrated.

Peripheral autonomic and somatic nervous system function can be compromised in chronic alcohol abuse (e.g. alcoholic polyneuropathy with variable reflex, sensory and motor dysfunction; orthostatic hypotension and hypothermia seen in Wernicke's encephalopathy). Pathological studies (Mayer and Garcia-Mullin 1972; Tredici and Minazzi 1975; Walsh and McLeod 1970) show axonal degeneration of myelinated and unmyelinated fibres, and demyelination. We have noted decreased bulbocavernosus (BC) activity and increased BC nerve conduction times in some of our alcoholic patients with impaired NPT.

Research is proceeding on ethanol's effects on neurotransmitter synthesis and turnover, cyclic nucleotide function (the 'second messengers' for some hormones and neurotransmitters), neuronal membrane integrity, receptor number, conformation and sensitivity, and other areas of neurophysiology. There is some evidence that chronic ethanol administration impairs or alters all of these systems, and recent reviews of the subject have been presented by Blum (1982) and Tabakoff (1977). These areas of research promise to yield much useful information on the mechanisms of alcohol-induced sexual and other neurophysiological dysfunction.

TREATMENT POSSIBILITIES

As in any disorder, the treatment should attempt to correct the underlying pathological process when possible. In alcohol-associated impotence, the patient should discontinue alcohol consumption at once. It is impossible to evaluate baseline and maximal erectile capacity while the patient continues to imbibe, and, of course, continued consumption can be expected to exacerbate the sexual dysfunction as well as any other concurrent psychiatric or medical illnesses.

A determination of probable aetiologic contributors to the impotence can be made by sleep laboratory NPT evaluation, including psychological testing, psychiatric interview, endocrine studies, and cardiovascular and neurological function studies. The procedure is described in full in Chapter 5. If an organic dysfunction is diagnosed, surgical intervention may be recommended, insertion of a penile prosthesis being the usual method used (Scott, Bradley and Timm 1973; Scott and Kantzavelos 1981). Arterial bypass may be used in certain cases of vascular insufficiency as revealed by arteriography, whilst a variety of treatment models and clinics exist for therapy of psychogenic impotence, when this is diagnosed (Masters and Johnson 1970; Meyer 1976).

CONCLUSIONS

That chronic alcoholics have impaired erectile function in comparison to healthy individuals has been suspected and subjectively reported. This study is the first systematic, objective verification of decreased erectile function. We found a decreased number and duration of maximum erections and increased number and duration of semi-erections, a pattern which we have seen in other types of organic impotence. Clearly more study needs to be undertaken, in terms of verification and extension of our findings. Detailed neurological, endocrinological, and vascular studies can help determine aetiologic factors in the erectile dysfunction. Future longitudinal studies can clarify prognosis and explore the possibility of some recovery of function with continued abstinence from ethanol.

References

Akhtar, M. J. (1977). Sexual disorders in male alcoholics. In *Alcoholism and drug dependence: a multidisciplinary approach* (eds. J. S. Madden, R. Walker and W. H. Kenyon. pp. 3–12. Plenum Press, New York.
Badr, F. M. and Bartke, A. (1974). Effect of ethyl alcohol on plasma testosterone level in mice. *Steroids* **23**, 921–8.
Blum, K. (1982). Neurophysiological effects of alcohol. In *Encyclopedic Handbook of Alcoholism* (eds. E. M. Pattison and E. Kaufman). Gardner Press, New York.
Bridell, D. W. and Wilson, J. T. (1976). Effects of alcohol and expectancy set on male sexual arousal. *J. Abnorm. Psychol.* **85**, 225–34.
Chapin, R. E., Breese, G. R., and Mueller, R. A. (1980). Possible mechanisms of reduction of plasma luteinizing hormone by ethanol. *J. Pharmacol. Exp. Ther.* **212**, 6–10.
Cicero, T. J. and Badger, T. M. (1977a). Effects of alcohol on the hypothalamic-pituitary-gonadal axis in the male rat. *J. Pharmacol. Exp. Ther.* **201**, 427–33.
—— —— (1977b). A comparative analysis of the effects of narcotics, alcohol and the barbiturates on the hypothalamic-pituitary-gonadal axis. *Adv. Exp. Med. Biol.* **85B**, 95–115.
—— Meyer, E. R., and Bell, R. D. (1979). Effects of alcohol on the hypothalmic-pituitary-luteinizing hormone axis and testicular steroidogenesis. *J. Pharmacol. Exp. Ther.* **208**, 210–15.

Cunningham, G. R., Karacan, I., Ware, J. C., Lantz, G. D., and Thornby, J. I. (1982). The relationship between serum testosterone and prolactin levels and nocturnal penile tumescence (NPT) in impotent men. *J. Androl.* **3**, 241–7.

Diagnostic and Statistical Manual of Mental Disorders, Third Edition, (1980). American Psychiatric Association, Washington, DC.

Farkas, G. M. and Rosen, R. C. (1976). Effect of alcohol on elicited male sexual response. *J. Stud. Alcohol.* **37**, 265–71.

Gantt, H. W. (1940). Effect of alcohol on sexual reflexes in dogs. *Am. J. Physiol.* **129**, 360–6.

—— (1952). Effects of alcohol on the sexual reflexes of normal and neurotic male dogs. *Psychosom. Med.* **14**, 174–81.

GAP Report No. 88, (1973). Assessment of sexual functioning: a guide to interviewing. *Group Adv. Psychiat.* **8**, 755–850.

Gordon, G. G., Altman, K., Southren, A. L., Rubin, E., and Lieber, C. S. (1976). Effect of alcohol (ethanol) administration on sex hormone metabolism in normal men. *N. Engl. J. Med.* **295**, 793–7.

—— and Southren, A. L. (1977). Metabolic effects of alcohol on the endocrine system. In *Metabolic Aspects of Alcoholism*, (ed. C. S. Lieber) pp. 249–302. University Park Press, Baltimore.

—— —— and Lieber, C. S. (1978). The effects of alcoholic liver disease and alcohol ingestion on sex hormones. *Alcoholism: Clin. Exp. Res.* **2**, 259–63.

Karacan, I. (1969). A simple and inexpensive transducer for quantitative measurement of penile tumescence during sleep. *Behav. Res. Meth. Instrum.* **2**, 251–52.

—— Salis, P. J., and Williams, R. L. (1978). The role of the sleep laboratory in diagnosis and treatment of impotence. In *Sleep disorders: diagnosis and treatment* (eds. R. L. Williams and I. Karacan). John Wiley, New York.

Lemere, F. and Smith, J. W. (1973). Alcohol-induced sexual impotence. *Am. J. Psychiatr.* **130**, 212–13.

Masters, W. H. and Johnson, V. E. (1970). *Human sexual inadequacy*, p. 160. Little, Brown, Boston.

Mayer, R., and Garcia-Mullin, R. (1972). Peripheral nerve and muscle disorders associated with alcoholism. In *The biology of alcoholism* (Vol. 2) (eds. B. Kassin and H. Begleiter). Plenum Press, New York.

Mendelson, J. H., Mello N. K., and Ellingboe, J. (1977). Effects of acute alcohol intake on pituitary-gonadal hormones in normal human males. *J. Pharmacol. Exp. Ther.* **202**, 676–82.

Meyer, J. K. (1976). *Clinical management of sexual disorders.* Williams and Wilkins, Baltimore.

National Council on Alcoholism criteria for the diagnosis of alcoholism. (1972). *Am. J. Psychiat.* **129**, 127–34.

Powell, B. J., Viamontes, J. A., and Brown, C. S. (1974). Alcohol effects on the sexual potency of alcoholic and non-alcoholic males. *Alcoholism, Zagreb* **10**, 78–80.

Rubin, H. B. and Henson, D. E. (1976). Effects of alcohol on male sexual responding. *Psychopharmacology* **47**, 123–34.

Scott, F. B., Bradley, W. E., and Timm, G. W. (1973). Management of erectile impotence: use of implantable inflatable prosthesis. *Urology* **2**, 80–2.

—— and Kantzavelos, D. A. (1981). Erectile impotence after urologic cancer surgery treated with the inflatable penile prosthesis. In *Sexual rehabilitation of the urologic cancer patient.* (eds. A. C. von Eschenback and D. B. Rodriguez. Hall, Boston.

Snyder, S. and Karacan, I. (1981). Effects of chronic alcoholism on nocturnal penile tumescence. *Psychosom. Med.* **43**, 423–9.

Tabakoff, B. (1977). Neurochemical aspects of ethanol dependence. In *Alcohol and Opiates: Neurochemical and Behavioral Mechanisms* (ed. K. Blum), Academic Press, New York.

Teitelbaum, H. A. and Gantt, W. H. (1958). The effect of alcohol on sexual reflexes sperm count in the dog. *Q. J. Stud. Alcohol* **19**, 394-8.

Tredici, G. and Minazzi, M. (1975). Alcoholic neuropathy: an electron microscopic study. *J. Neurol. Sci.* **25**, 33-346.

Van Thiel, D. H., Gavaler, J. S., Lester, R., Loriaux, D. L., and Braunstein, J. D. (1975). Plasma estrone, prolactin, neurophysin, and sex steroid-binding globulin in chronic alcoholic men. *Metabolism* **24**, 1015-19.

— — Lester, R., and Vaitukaitis, J. (1978). Evidence for a defect in pituitary secretion of luteinizing hormone in chronic alcoholic men. *J. Clin. Endocrinol. Metab.* **47**, 499-507.

Walsh, J. and McLeod, J. (1970). Alcoholic neuropathy: an electrophysiological and histological study. *J. Neurol. Sci.* **10**, 457-69.

Whalley, L. J. (1973). Sexual adjustment of male alcoholics. *Acta Psychiat. Scand.* **58**, 281-98.

Williams, R. L., Agnew, H. W., and Webb, W. B. (1964). Sleep patterns in young adults: an EEG study. *Electroencephalogr. Clin. Neurophysiol.* **17**, 376-81.

— — Karacan, I., and Hursch, C. J. (1974). *Electroencephalography of human sleep: clinical applications.* John Wiley, New York.

Wright, J., Merry, J., Fry, D., and Marks, V. (1976). Pituitary function in chronic alcoholism. In *Alcohol intoxication and withdrawal* (ed. M. M. Gross) pp. 253-6. *Adv. Exp. Med. Biol.*, Vol. 59. Plenum Press, New York.

Ylikahri, R. H., Huttunen, M. O., Harkonen, M., Leino, T., Helenius, T., Liewendahl, K., and Karonen, S. L. (1978). Acute effects of alcohol on anterior pituitary secretion of the tropic hormones. *J. Clin. Endocrinol. Metab.* **46**, 715-20.

Sex and drugs

10

Cholinergic and adrenergic control of human sexual responses

ALAN J. RILEY AND ELIZABETH J. RILEY

INTRODUCTION

THE SEXUAL RESPONSE depends upon the integrity of the autonomic nervous system. A triphasic model of autonomic nervous system activation has been proposed to account for the sequential nature of the sexual response (Wegner, Jones, and Jones 1956). Parasympathetic nervous system activation occurs first and dominates the initial phases of sexual arousal. With increasing sexual stimulation there is progressive activation of the sympathetic nervous system, and at the time of ejaculation (and orgasm) the sympathetic nervous system dominates. After orgasm, parasympathetic nervous activity again becomes dominant until the autonomic nervous system returns to its pre-arousal level. Acceptance of this model implies that the physiological changes that characterize the early stages of sexual arousal are dependent upon parasympathetic nervous stimulation.

It is commonly stated that erection is initiated by cholinergic impulses (Bell 1972; Kaplan 1974a; Weiss 1972). By analogy it is proposed that sexual arousal in the female, characterised by vaginal lubrication and vasocongestion, is also stimulated by cholinergic impulses (Kaplan 1974b). Although drugs possessing anticholinergic activity may impair sexual arousal (Horowitz and Goble, 1979; Medical Letter 1977, 1980; Renshaw 1978), the evidence to support this statement is very weak and is derived essentially from the reported occurrence of erectile dysfunction during treatment with drugs possessing anticholinergic activity. Certainly, the number of patients complaining of erectile difficulties during treatment with such drugs is very small, relative to their extensive use.

CHOLINERGIC AGONISTS AND ANTAGONISTS

Animal studies have demonstrated the dependence of sexual behaviour upon cholinergic stimulation, and impairment of sexual function by anticholinergic drugs (Bignami 1956; Singer 1968). Atropine administered to male rats during coitus abolished all elements of sexual behaviour very quickly, whilst nicotine (0.6 mg/kg) facilitated all components of male sexual function (Soulairac and Soulairac 1975). Human sexual arousal has not been reported to be initiated or facilitated by cholinergic agonists, although injection of acetylcholine into the septal region of the brain of an epileptic female patient resulted in euphoria and sexual arousal often culminating in repetitive orgasms (Heath 1972). It is not known whether this response occurs in non-epileptic subjects.

Effects of atropine

The effect of atropine on human sexual function has been studied in male and female volunteers. In six out of seven men, intravenous administration of atropine (0.035 mg/kg) did not influence erectile function, determined by penile plethysmography, whether the subjects were stimulated visually or by vibration (Wagner and Brindley 1980). The same dose of atropine was given to a group of six female subjects prior to masturbation, during which vaginal blood flow was monitored by hot film anemometry (Wagner and Levin 1980). The heart rate was monitored to confirm that blockade of the muscarinic innervation of the heart had occurred. Clear evidence was obtained in all subjects of an increase in vaginal blood flow on initiation of masturbation culminating in orgasm, indicative of a normal sexual response. However, subjective assessment of the sexual response by the subjects themselves gave interesting results. One subject thought that she had to work harder to obtain her orgasm, and another subject found that atropine gave her a dry mouth and this made her breathing during sexual arousal more difficult than usual. Her sexual arousal kept falling off despite the use of a vibrator and she had a poor quality orgasm, after which she still felt full and tense in the vagina, features only usually present when her orgasmic release was poor.

In another study by the same investigators, five women were each given methylatropine, 1 mg orally, 4 h and 1 h before sexual activity. Two subjects felt that this treatment resulted in prolongation of the time required to induce orgasm by masturbation (Wagner and Levin 1980). The study, however, was uncontrolled. Nevertheless the results of these studies suggest that atropine may adversely affect the attainment and quality of orgasm in females, rather than impair initial sexual arousal, as would have been expected from the literature.

Female volunteers

We have studied the effect of cholinergic stimulation and atropine on the sexual response of female volunteers. Each of six subjects was studied on three occasions during a single menstrual cycle. The experiments were conducted on days 6, 9, and 12 of the menstrual cycle, each time within the period 24–36 h after the subject's previous orgasmic experience. The subject took a coded treatment orally (either two bethanechol (25 mg) tablets or two matching placebo tablets) at 18.00 h. At this time she inserted a vaginal tampon. At 19.45 hours the subject attended the experimental room and after resting for 10 min her pulse rate was measured. Atropine (1.5 mg) or saline was then given by slow intravenous injection and after a further 10 min the pulse rate was again recorded. The vaginal tampon was removed and replaced with two tampons, and a wad of absorbant wool was placed at the introitus between the labia, after wiping the vulva dry. The wad of wool and the vaginal tampons were pre-weighed separately. The subject then proceeded to masturbate by means of a standard vibrator, the time taken to reach orgasm was recorded by the subjects by means of a blinded stop clock. Following orgasm the subject completed standard rating scales for the assessment of the subjective features of the sexual response (Fig. 10.1). They also commented on side effects. The tampons and wad of wool were removed, placed in sealed polythene bags and reweighed.

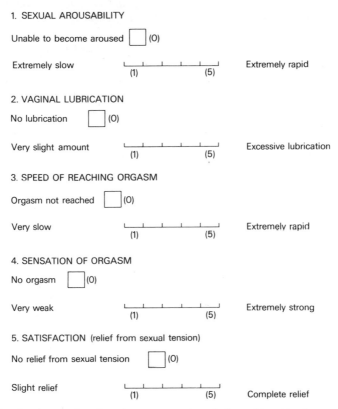

FIG 10.1   Rating scales for the assessment of the subjective features of the sexual response.

The treatments were arranged so that each subject received the following:
(a) Placebo tablets, saline injection.
(b) Placebo tablets, atropine injection.
(c) Bethanechol tablets, saline injection.
The order of treatment administration relative to the menstrual day was randomized according to a predetermined Latin square arrangement.

Results of cholinergic stimulation

All subjects completed the study. Following atropine there was a significant increase in pulse rate from 77 ± 7 to 107 ± 13 b.p.m. (mean ± SD), but there was no change in heart rate after bethanechol. The median (range) weights of genital secretion absorbed by the tampons (vaginal, also including secretion from the cervical canal) and wad of wool (vulval) and the times taken to reach orgasm are given in Table 10.1. No significant differences were recorded between the treatments for weight of genital secretion, or for the time taken to reach orgasm.

TABLE 10.1 *Median (range) for weight of genital secretion and time to orgasm in six subjects after placebo, atropine, and bethanechol*

	Placebo	Atropine	Bethanechol
Genital secretion, total (g)	2.15 (0.88–4.43)	2.49 (1.89–4.16)	2.615 (1.82–4.75)
Genital secretion, vaginal (g)	1.355 (0.40–2.27)	1.455 (1.08–2.22)	1.39 (0.34–2.91)
Genital secretion, vulval (g)	0.83 (0.48–2.16)	0.56 (0.38–2.82)	1.47 (0.63–1.98)
Time to orgasm (min)	5.3 (3.9–9.1)	5.95 (4.3–11.8)	4.85 (3.7–7.4)

The median (range) self-rating scores for the subjective features of the sexual response are shown in Table 10.2. There were no differences among the treatments for arousability, sensation of orgasm, and satisfaction. The differences between the treatments for speed of reaching orgasm just failed to reach a level of statistical significance (P = 0.052).

TABLE 10.2 *Median (range) self-rating scores for subjective features of sexual response after placebo, atropine, and bethanechol in six female subjects*

Feature	Placebo	Atropine	Bethanechol
Arousability	3(3–4)	3(2–5)	3(2–5)
Speed to orgasm	3(2–4)	2(1–3)	3.5(2–5)
Sensation of orgasm	3(2–5)	3(2–4)	4(3–5)
Satisfaction	3.5(2–5)	2(1–3)	3.5(2–4)

Five subjects complained of visual disturbances following atropine and all six subjects complained of a dry mouth. Two subjects complained of palpitations after atropine. One subject reported headache after placebo, and following bethanechol three subjects complained of nausea and one of these also complained of abdominal pain and urinary frequency. These side effects can be explained by cholinergic stimulation and therefore confirm that the drug was having a pharmacological effect.

To ensure that the time of the menstrual cycle on which the different treatments were given did not influence the time taken to reach orgasm nor the weight of genital secretion, these data were reclassified according to the day of menstrual cycle, irrespective of the treatment given. The median and ranges of the parameters measured, classified by the day of cycle are given in Table 10.3. No differences existed between the menstrual days for either weight of genital secretion (total, vulval, and vaginal) or time to orgasm.

TABLE 10.3 *Median and range for weight of genital secretion and time to orgasm, classified according to day of menstrual cycle.*

	Day 6	Day 9	Day 12
Genital secretion, total (g)	2.25 (0.88–4.16)	2.265 (1.45–4.43)	2.86 (1.95–4.75)
Genital secretion, vaginal (g)	1.075 (0.34–1.71)	1.52 (0.83–2.27)	1.74 (1.06–2.91)
Genital secretion, vulval (g)	1.18 (0.48–2.82)	0.685 (0.42–2.16)	1.065 (0.38–1.98)
Time to orgasm (min)	6.55 (4.0–9.1)	4.85 (3.7–11.8)	5.55 (4.3–6.4)

The self-report rating scales used in this study have been used fairly extensively in other studies and have been found to be capable of picking up changes in sexual response. Studies undertaken to validate the rating scales will form the basis of another publication.

The results of this study suggest that sexual arousal, in particular genital lubrication and orgasm, are not dependant upon muscarinic cholinergic mechanisms. The antihistaminic drug, brompheniramine, possesses anticholinergic activity and has been used in the treatment of retrograde ejaculation (Andaloro and Dube 1975; Budd 1975). It has been postulated that in diabetic retrograde ejaculation, there is diminished sympathetic input to the smooth muscle of the bladder neck, which results in dominance of the parasympathetic stimulation of this tissue, which would prevent closure of the bladder neck. The administration of an anticholinergic drug should restore the balance of autonomic nervous system stimulation. However, injection of atropine prior to masturbation in a diabetic patient suffering from retrograde ejaculation, did not improve ejaculatory efficiency (personal observation).

ADRENERGIC CONTROL MECHANISMS

According to the triphasic model of autonomic nervous system activation described above, sympathetic activity dominates the later stages of the sexual response. There is both biochemical and physiological evidence of increased sympathetic activity during sexual arousal. A significant correlation has been found between stages of sexual arousal, erection quality, and plasma noradrenaline concentration in a male subject (Wiedeking, Lake, Ziegler, Kowarski, and Money 1979). In a second study (Wiedeking, Ziegler, and Wake 1979), changes in plasma concentration of noradrenaline and dopamine betahydroxylase during coitus, were monitored in two men and two women. In all subjects increasing sexual arousal was associated with an increase in plasma noradrenaline level, the greatest increases occurring when sexual arousal resulted in orgasm. Percentage change in plasma dopamine β-hydroxylase concentration significantly correlated with the plasma concentration of noradrenaline. Following orgasm there was a rapid decrease in plasma noradrenaline level, an observation that is compatible with the triphasic model.

Physiological evidence for activation of the sympathetic nervous system during sexual response is provided by the extragenital changes that accompany it. These become most evident during the plateau phase of the sexual response (Masters and Johnson 1966), and sexual arousal is associated with an increase in blood pressure in both sexes. During psychogenically induced sexual arousal to orgasm, an increase in systolic blood pressure of 50 mm Hg has been reported in women (Klumbies and Kleinsorge 1950). Increases in systolic and diastolic blood pressure of up to 100 mm Hg and 48 mm Hg respectively were found by intra-arterial blood pressure monitoring during coitus (Little, Honour, and Sleight 1974) and in this study a relative slowing of the heart at a time when the blood pressure was rising was reported. Such cardiovascular events occur when noradrenaline is infused into healthy volunteers (Richards, Prichard, and Hernandez 1979).

Effects of adrenergic antagonism

Studies have been undertaken to determine the effect of antagonizing sympathetic stimulation at peripheral adrenoceptors. Preliminary data on the effects of orally administered propranolol and phenoxybenzamine on human penile erection as assessed by penile plethysmography, have been reported by Wagner and Brindley (1980). The study was qualitative in nature and sexual arousal was induced by visual stimulation and by vibration. Propranolol in doses of up to 120 mg for 2 days, did not cause disturbances in erection or ejaculation, in the three men studied. Phenoxybenzamine in doses from 40 to 120 mg daily, caused failure of ejaculation without impairing erection. It is not stated whether the subjects experienced the sensation of orgasm.

Single oral dosing with propranolol (160 mg) in two subjects 90 min before coitus, did not influence the subjective features of the sexual response, although it reduced the usual increase in blood pressure occurring at orgasm (Fox 1970). More recently, we have compared a single oral dose of propranolol (80 mg) and labetalol (100 mg), with placebo control, on the pressor response to sexual arousal induced by masturbation in six female volunteers (Riley and Riley 1981). Labetalol is an effective antihypertensive agent that acts by concurrent antagonism at α- and β-andrenoceptors. In this study labetalol, but not propranolol, significantly reduced the increase in blood pressure that occurred at orgasm. Since the dose of propranolol used had a greater β-blocking activity than labetalol, evidence is provided from this experiment for an α-receptor mediated mechanism, to account for the normal pressor response of sexual arousal. The subjective features of the sexual response were assessed by each subject using visual analogue scales. Subjects reported a significant reduction in vaginal lubrication with labetalol compared to both placebo and propranolol, but no other features of the sexual response were significantly altered by either treatment.

Experiments with labetalol

In view of the apparent effect of labetalol on vaginal lubrication found in this study, we have undertaken a more detailed investigation. Six female volunteers were each studied on three occasions (on days 6, 9, and 12), during a single menstrual cycle. The procedure was similar to that described in which the effect of atropine and bethanechol was investigated. There were, however, two major differences. Only total genital secretion (i.e. tampon and wad of cotton wool weighed collectively) was measured, and the orgasmic and post-orgasmic blood pressures were recorded as previously described. The treatments used were placebo and two doses of labetalol (100 mg and 300 mg), administered double-blind.

A dose-related inhibition of the orgasmic-pressure response was seen, but although labetalol was without discernible effect on the weight of genital secretion collected, there was a significant dose-related effect on the time taken to reach orgasm (Table 10.4). As the dose of labetalol increased so the time taken to reach orgasm increased. The time taken to reach orgasm was also assessed subjectively by the subjects on the standard rating scales (Figure 10.1) immediately following each experimental session. Significant differences were found between treatments for the scores for 'speed to orgasm', which decreased as the dose of labetalol increased. There was, therefore, good agreement between the subjective assessment of speed of attaining orgasm and the actual real time taken as measured by the clock. No differences between the treatments existed for the distribution of scores for arousability, sensation of orgasm, or satisfaction.

TABLE 10.4 *Genital secretion weights, time taken to reach orgasm, and subjective rating scales, in six female subjects after placebo and two doses of labetalol (100 mg, 300 mg), expressed as median (range)*

	Placebo	Labetalol (100 mg)	Labetalol (300 mg)
Weight secretion (g)	2.25 (1.62–2.86)	1.78 (1.01–4.34)	2.23 (0.94–2.99)
Time to orgasm (min)*	6.2 (4.2–10.3)	6.9 (5.5–12.8)	9.2 (5.1–12.3)
Subjective scores:			
Arousability	3 (2–4)	3 (3)	3.5 (2–4)
Speed to orgasm*	3 (2–4)	2.5 (1–4)	1.5 (1–2)
Sensation of orgasm	2.5 (2–4)	3 (2–4)	2.5 (2–4)
Satisfaction	3 (1–4)	3 (2–5)	4 (2–5)

*Significant ($P < 0.05$) dose-related effect.

The finding of labetalol-induced reduction in genital secretion assessed subjectively in the earlier study, was not confirmed by the objective measurements in the second study. Interestingly it has been reported that vaginal secretion decreases with prolonged sexual arousal (Masters and Johnson 1966) and therefore the subjective reduction in secretion reported in the first study, may have been caused by labetalol delaying orgasm. However, this was not apparent on the results of the analogue rating scale for 'speed to orgasm', reported in that study. The inaccuracies of this type of subjective assessment in small subject groups is well recognized and it is for this reason that we have adopted the ordinal rating scale in subsequent work.

The effect of labetalol on male sexual response has also been studied (Riley, Riley, and Davies 1982). Penile plethysmographic recording of the sexual response, culminating in ejaculation, was undertaken after treatment with two doses (100 mg and 300 mg) labetalol and placebo, in each of six male volunteers. Labetalol did not influence the attainment or maintenance of erection, but it did however cause a significant dose-related delay in ejaculation (Figure 10.2). Labetalol also delayed the process of detumescence in a dose-related manner (Figure 10.3) and this latter observation is interesting in that it lends support to the hypothesis that detumescence results from sympathetic stimulation (Kuntz 1953), which would be blocked by labetalol, probably by its α-adrenoceptor

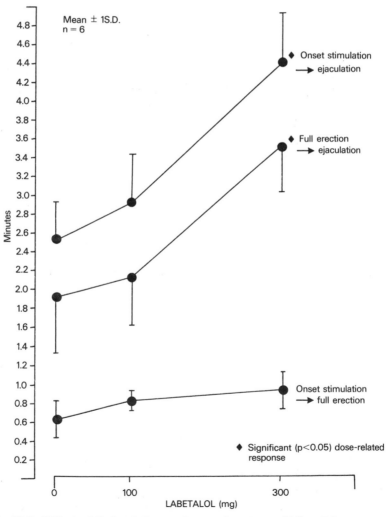

FIG. 10.2 Effect of Labetalol on male sexual response (Riley, Riley, and Davies 1982).

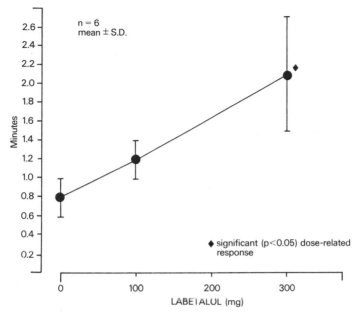

FIG. 10.3 Effect of Labetalol on detumescence (Riley, Riley, and Davies 1982).

antagonist activity. Priapism has been reported to occur in association with treatment with drugs that exhibit α-adrenoceptor antagonist activity (Bhalla, Hoffbrand and Phatak 1979; Law 1980), including chlorpromazine (Bourgeois 1972; Meiraz and Fishelvitch 1967).

Failure of ejaculation

Many psychoactive drugs have been reported to cause delayed ejaculation or failure of ejaculation and to inhibit female orgasm. This raises a question of terminology. Failure of ejaculation should only be used when the male experiences orgasm but this is not accompanied by ejaculation. In one study (Blair and Simpson 1966), a drug was said to cause 'total interference' with ejaculation, if no ejaculate was produced in a time of at least double the patients' normal time to achieve ejaculation. This is clearly an unsatisfactory definition since in the labetalol study alluded to previously, the time taken for some subjects to reach ejaculation after labetalol was greater than twofold that required after placebo.

Some authors have postulated that the failure of ejaculation associated with the use of antipsychotic agents is mediated by their peripheral adrenergic blocking activity (Shader 1964). It has also been suggested that these drugs cause preorgasmic detumescence of the glans since, in men who complain of absent or delayed orgasm, the glans is said to be flaccid even when erection is complete (Comfort 1979). This may well be the case in some men but it is not a universal observation. Of nine patients we have seen on account of drug-induced failure of ejaculation (and failure or orgasm in two cases), none experienced premature detumescence of the glans, as determined by their own subjective assessment.

Whilst it may seem reasonable to explain the delay in ejaculation induced by α-adrenoceptor antagonists in terms of peripheral mechanisms, a central effect cannot be completely dismissed. The neurohypophyseal hormones may be involved in the physiology of ejaculation and orgasm but circulating levels of oxytocin are increased in relation to ejaculation (Ogawa, Kudo, Kitsuno, and Fukuchi 1980) and orgasm in the female (Fox and Knaggs 1969). Alpha-adrenoceptors are stimulatory to the central control of the milk ejection reflex (i.e. release of oxytocin) in the rat (Tribollet, Clarke, Dreifuss, and Lincoln 1978). Alpha-adrenoceptor antagonists may therefore inhibit the secretion of oxytocin. What is not known at the present time is the exact role of oxytocin in the physiology of ejaculation and orgasm. Many women are unable to experience orgasm without nipple stimulation, an observation which may provide evidence that increased oxytocin secretion is important in the initiation of orgasm.

Effects of adrenergic stimulation

If α-adrenoceptor antagonism results in delayed ejaculation and orgasm, can the converse effect be obtained by the use of α-adrenoceptor agonists? Midodrine, a selective α-adrenoceptor agonist,* given intravenously in a dose of 5 mg failed to significantly influence the time taken for a group of six female volunteers to reach orgasm, under controlled conditions (personal observation). This treatment did result in a significant increase in blood pressure, confirming that the midodrine was exerting a pharmacological effect, but there was no significant effect on the subjective features of the sexual response. However, five of the six subjects ranked 'arousability' less after midodrine than after placebo. Studies are underway investigating the effect of α-adrenoceptor stimulation on sexual function in male volunteer subjects and preliminary results indicate that intravenous midodrine inhibited erection in three out of five men studied.

Retrograde ejaculation

Drugs possessing α-adrenergic agonist activity have been used with success in the treatment of retrograde ejaculation. Ephedrine (50 mg orally) taken 1-2 h before intercourse was the first drug to be used for this purpose (Stewart and Bergant 1974). With the use of phenylpropanolamine, restoration of normal ejaculation was achieved in one patient with retrograde ejaculation, due to diabetes. Phenylpropanolamine was also used to treat six patients with retrograde ejaculation, of whom four responded favourably (Sandler 1979). The four patients who did respond to this treatment were diagnosed as having idiopathic retrograde ejaculation, while the two failures had organic disease.

A therapeutic trial of intravenously administered phenylephrine, administered 1 h before masturbation, was conducted in a group of six men who had partial or complete loss of ejaculation after retroperitoneal lymphadenectomy (Stockamp, Schreiter, and Altwein 1974). Before therapy, four patients were unable to ejaculate and two produced a diminished almost azoospermatic ejaculate. With one exception, retrograde ejaculation was not present, suggesting a diagnosis of impairment of emission. The administration of phenylephrine further impaired antegrade ejaculation in the two patients who had a diminished ejaculate, whilst in three patients the loss of ejaculation persisted, and the urinary sperm counts in all these five patients showed further decrease relative to pretreatment counts. Only the patient with diagnosed retrograde ejaculation was able to experience antegrade ejaculation following treatment. The authors concluded that α-adrenoceptor agonists are ineffective in correcting impairment of the emissive phase of the ejaculatory response. This may not be the case. The selective α-adrenoceptor agonist, midodrine, has been found useful in the treatment of ejaculatory disorders following retroperitoneal lymphadenectomy (Jones, Linzbach, and Weber 1979).

Actions of midodrine

The effect of midodrine in the treatment of partial ejaculatory incompetence has been evaluated (Riley and Riley 1982). This is an interesting form of sexual dysfunction in which the patients' main complaint is lack of orgasmic sensation. The semen in these patients is not forcibly ejaculated but instead dribbles from the urethral meatus. Kaplan (1974c) feels that this condition is frequently psychogenic and responds favourably to psychotherapy, but we have been disappointed by this therapeutic approach. Masters (cited by Kaplan 1974c) considers that partial ejaculatory incompetence is often due to organic factors which interfere with the filling of the posterior urethral bulb with semen, during the emission phase of the ejaculatory process. Treatment with midodrine resulted in a significant improvement in orgasmic sensation but did not influence the time taken to achieve ejaculation as assessed subjectively. The improvement in orgasmic sensation was associated with improved ejaculatory efficiency in five of the six patients studied, but the treatment period in this study was only 10 days. In a further evaluation of midodrine in this condition, the drug was given for 6 weeks, following a 2-week placebo run-in period. During the fourth week of treatment with midodrine there was a significant reduction in the time taken to attain ejaculation. The beneficial effect of the drug on orgasmic sensation observed in the earlier experiment, was confirmed (personal observation). These observations provide further evidence of the dependence of the ejaculatory process on α-adrenoceptor stimulation.

CONCLUSIONS

As many as 30 per cent of patients presenting with sexual difficulties are found to have an organic abnormality, although at the present time it is not always possible to make a definite association between a diagnosed organic disturbance and the presenting sexual problem. This incidence of organic abnormality is higher than is generally recognized, and probably accounts for the relatively high failure rate of the psychotherapeutic approach to sexual problems. A greater understanding of the physiology of sexual function and the neurotransmitters involved in the sexual response, may suggest new pharmacotherapeutic approaches to the management of sexual dysfunction.

References

Andaloro, V. A. and Dube, A. (1975). Treatment of retrograde ejaculation with brompheniramine. *Urology* **5**, 520-2.

Bell, C. (1972). Autonomic nervous control of reproduction: circulatory and other factors. *Pharmacol. Rev.* **24**, 657-736.

Bhalla, A. K., Hoffbrand, B. I., and Phatak, P. S. (1979). Prazosin and priapism. *Br. Med. J.* **ii**, 1039.

Bignami, G. (1966). Pharamcologic influences on mating behaviour in the male rat. Effects of *d*-amphetamine, LSD-25, Strychnine, nicotine and various anticholinergic agents. *Psychopharmacologia* **10**, 44-58.

Blair, J. H. and Simpson, G. M. (1966). Effect of antipsychotic drugs on reproductive functions. *Dis. Nerv. Syst.* **27**, 645-7.

Bourgeois, M. (1972). Priapismes sous neuroceptique (trois cas). *Nouve. Presse Med.* **1**, 161.

Budd, H. A. (1975). Brompheniramine in treatment of retrograde ejaculation. *Urology* **6**, 131.

Comfort, A. (1979). Effects of psychoactive drugs on ejaculation. *Am. J. Psychiat.* **136**, 124-5.

Fox, C. (1970). Reduction in the rise of systolic blood pressure during human coitus by the beta-adrenergic blocking agent, propranolol. *J. Reprod. Fertil.* **22**, 587-90.

—— and Knaggs, G. S. (1969). Milk ejection activity (oxytocin) in peripheral venous blood in man during lactation and in association with coitus. *J. Endocrinol.* **45**, 145-6.

Heath, R. G. (1972). Pleasure and brain activity in man. *J. Nerv. Ment. Dis.* **154**, 3-00.

Horowitz, J. D. and Goble, A. J. (1979). Drugs and impaired male sexual function. *Drugs* **18**, 206-17.

Jonas, D., Linzbach, P., and Weber, W. (1979). The use of midodrine in the treatment of ejaculation disorders following retroperitoneal lymphadenectomy. *Eur. Urol.* **5**, 184-7.

Kaplan, H. S. (1974*a*). *The new sex therapy*, p. 86. Baillière Tindall, London.

—— (1974*b*). *The new sex therapy*, p. 87. Baillière Tindall, London.

—— (1974*c*). *The new sex therapy*, p. 319. Baillière Tindall, London.

Klumbies, G. and Kleinsorge, M. (1950). Circulatory changes and prophylaxis during orgasm. *Int. J. Sex.* **4**, 61-9.

Kuntz, A. (1953). *The autonomic nervous system*, pp. 295-6. 4th Edition. Lea-Febiger, Philadelphia.

Law, M. R., Copland, R. F. P., Armitstead, J. G., and Gabriel, R. (1980). Labetalol and priapism. *Br. Med. J.* **280**, 115.

Littler, W. A., Honour, A. J., and Sleight, P. (1974). Direct arterial pressure, heart rate and electrocardiogram during human coitus. *J. Reprod. Fertil.* **40**, 321-31.

Masters, W. and Johnson, V. E. (1966). *Human sexual response*. Little Brown, Boston.

Medical Letter, (1977). Clonidine (Catapres) and other drugs causing sexual dysfunction. *Med. Lett.* **19**, 81-2.

Medical Letter (1980). Drugs that cause sexual dysfunction. *Med. Lett.* **22**, 108-10.

Meiraz, D. and Fishelvitch, J. (1967). Priapism and largectal medication. *Israel J. Med. Sci.* **5**, 1254-5.

Ogawa, S., Kudo, S., Kitsunai, Y., and Fukuchi, S. (1980). Increase in oxytocin secretion at ejaculation in male. *Clin. Endocrinol.* **13**, 95-7.

Renshaw, D. C. (1978). Sex and drugs. *S.A. Med. J.* **54**, 322-6.

Richards, D. A., Prichard, B. N. C., and Hernandez, R. (1979). Circulatory effects of noradrenaline and adrenaline before and after labetalol. *Br. J. Clin. Pharmacol.* **7**, 371–8.

Riley, A. J. and Riley, E. J. (1982). The effect of labetalol and propranolol on the pressor response to sexual arousal in women. *Br. J. Clin. Pharmacol.* **12**, 341–4.

— — (1982). Partial ejaculatory incompetence in the therapeutic effect of midodrine, an orally active alpha-adrenoceptor agonist. *Eur. Urol.* **8**, 155–60.

— — and Davies, H. J. (1982). A method for monitoring drug effects of male sexual response on the effect of single dose labetalol. *Br. J. Clin. Pharmac.* **14**, 695–700.

Sandler, B. (1979). Idiopathic retrograde ejaculation. *Fertil. Steril.* **32**, 474–5.

Shader, R. I. (1964). Sexual dysfunction associated with thioridazine hydrochloride. *JAMA* **188**, 1007–9.

Singer, J. J. (1968). The effects of atropine upon the female and male sexual behaviour of rats. *Physiol. Behav.* **3**, 377–8.

Soulairac, M. C. and Soulairac, A. (1975). *Monoaminergic and cholinergic control of sexual behaviour; pharmacology and biochemistry* (eds. M. Sandler and G. L. Gessa) ppp. 99–116. Raven Press, New York.

Stewart, B. H. and Bergant, J. A. (1974). Correction of retrograde ejaculation by sympathomimetic medication: preliminary report. *Fertil. Steril.* **25**, 1073–4.

Stockamp, K., Schreiter, F., and Altwein, J. E. (1974). Alpha-adrenergic drugs in retrograde ejaculation. *Fertil. Steril.* **25**, 817–20.

Tribollet, E., Clarke, G., Dreifuss, J. J., and Lincoln, D. W. (1978). The rate of central adrenergic receptors in the reflex release of oxytocin. *Brain Res.* **142**, 69–84.

Wagner, G. and Brindley, G. S. (1980). The effect of atropine and alpha- and beta-blockers on human penile erection: A controlled study. In *First International Conference on Vascular Impotence* (Ed. A. Zorgniotti). Thomas, New York.

Wagner, G., and Levin, R. J. (1980). Effect of atropine and methylatropine on human vaginal blood flow, sexual arousal and climax. *Acta. Pharmac. Toxicol.* **46**. 321–5.

Wegner, M. A., Jones, F. N., and Jones, M. H. (1956). *Physiological physiology*. Holt, New York.

Weiss, H. D. (1972). The physiology of human erection. *Ann. Int. Med.* **76**, 793–9.

Wiedeking, C., Lake, C. R., Ziegler, M., Kowarski, A. A., and Money, J. (1979). Plasma noradrenaline and dopamine beta-hydroxylase during sexual activity. *Psychosom. Med.* **39**, 143–8.

Wiedeking, C., Ziegler, M. G., and Lake, C. R. (1979). Plasma noradrenaline and dopamine beta-hydroxylase during human sexual activity. *J. Psychiat. Res.* **15**, 139–45.

We appreciate the careful secretarial work undertaken by Kim Costen in the preparation of this manuscript. We are grateful to the following companies for the supply of drugs: Chemie Linz AG (midodrine); Glenwood Laboratories Ltd (bethanechol); Glaxo Group Research Ltd, Ware (labetalol and propranolol).

11

Sexual dysfunction and prescribed psychotropic drugs

JOHN M. H. REES

DRUG INDUCED sexual dysfunction has only attracted publicity in recent years. Amongst the many difficulties encountered are those relating to the incidence of such dysfunctions, and the mechanisms by which they occur. This short review concentrates on these two difficulties in the context of iatrogenic sexual dysfunction caused by psychotropic drugs. Recent reviews of all aspects of drug induced sexual dysfunction include those of Horowitz and Goble (1979), Millar (1979), Seagraves (1979), and Griffin (1981). Helpful summaries also appear in successive editions of Dukes' Side Effects of Drugs Annual.

EVALUATING THE PROBLEM

A major difficulty in the past has been one of looseness of terminology, and, up to a point, this persists. For instance 'impotence' (in the male) has been used to describe absence of erection, failure of ejaculation, or even lack of interest. Since drugs can have an effect on each of these components, in this chapter an attempt has been made to identify the precise nature of the dysfunction.

Quantitative data is difficult to obtain for several reasons. Apart from the obvious complexity of the physiological and psychological control of these emotions and reflexes, the next problem is the difficulty in distinguishing between the disease state and the effect of the drug. A good example is the lack of sexual interest that characterizes depression and the well-documented erectile failure caused by antidepressant drugs.

A third problem is the greater than average reluctance to admit to sexual inadequacy, particularly by the male population. A side effect may only be admitted if it is specifically requested and this then compounds the problem. In healthy drug-free individuals, sexual dissatisfaction is not uncommon. Masters and Johnson estimated it in 20 per cent of marriages. It is clear then that a specific request concerning a side effect may elicit an answer leading to a false conclusion of a causal relationship.

For instance, in 1972 Wheatley enquired whether the then new neuroleptic drug thioridazine had been reported as disturbing sexual function in a general practitioner clinical trial (G.P. Research Group 1972). It had not, nor did the authors feel that it had occurred. Yet 4 years later following a trial in which specific questions were asked, after admittedly some higher doses, the incidence of sexual dysfunction in males with this drug was rated as high as 60 per cent (Kotin, Wilbert, Verburg, and Soldinger 1976). The reported incidence of impotence due to methyldopa ranges from 0.1 to 25 per cent, depending on how the information is gleaned (Horowitz and Goble 1979), and that due to tricyclic antidepressants from 0.5 per cent (Beaumont 1973) to over 70 per cent (Couper-Smartt and Rodham 1973).

A further problem is that a sexual side effect of a drug may appear in the literature following a single observation, and, despite extensive attempts at confirmation, may persist in the literature. Good examples are 'aphrodisia' caused by mazindol (Friesen 1976), and 'ejaculatory failure' caused by chlordiazepoxide (Hughes 1964). Next is the possibility that a side effect may not be reported because it is not deemed 'unwanted'. It is difficult to imagine a circumstance in which drug-induced aphrodisia would consistently be reported to the general practitioner, though presumably word would spread. Equally there may be instances in which decreased libido would seem heaven sent by at least one partner. Couper-Smartt and Rodham (1973) stressed that '. . . not all patients felt the (sexual) symptoms represented difficulties . . .'.

Then there is the unique difficulty of experimentation. Clinical trials are difficult to control, and volunteer trials, whilst making fascinating reading, do raise the question as to whether the supreme dedication and calibre of the volunteers can possibly enable them to be described as representative of the general population. Lastly, it follows that the greater the number of drugs taken, the greater the incidence of side effects. Drug intake tends to increase with years, during which time other organic disorders and hormonal factors may contribute to sexual dysfunction (e.g. hypertension) which is then erroneously associated with the drug.

DRUGS ACTING ON THE CNS

A brief summary of the actions of some centrally-acting drugs follows (and it is by no means comprehensive), in which emphasis is placed on the major targets for drug-induced sexual dysfunction. These are: effects on libido in either sex; interference with the autonomic control of erection and ejaculation in the male; an effect on female orgasm (about which so little is known), and an action mediated via hormones, notably in the release mechanisms of prolactin and luteinizing hormone.

The old pharmacological distinction between stimulants, antidepressants, neuroleptics, and anxiolytics/sedatives is employed. It is worth stressing that this distinction is only currently one of convenience and will soon lose any pharmacological or psychiatric relevance as new drugs are developed that differ so clearly from original prototypes.

Sympathomimetic anorectic agents

Garattini (1980) has differentiated between anorectics that release catecholamines (amphetamine, diethylpropion, mazindol), and those that release 5-hydroxytryptamine (fenfluramine), though in the opinion of this reviewer the distinction is not quite so clear cut.

One would anticipate that amphetamine would have prominent effects on sexual function, if only because of its well-known euphoriant action (like cocaine, for instance) which has been likened to orgasm. In addition, amphetamine releases dopamine (and is probably as potent a dopaminergic agonist as any) and there is potential interference with hypothalamic and endocrinological function. Amphetamine is recorded in the literature as causing gynaecomastia (Tooley and Lack, 1949), surprising though that may seem, since it is the dopamine antagonists that are commonly associated with this side effect. In addition, the whole problem is compounded since gynaecomastia may be difficult to identify in someone who is overweight. On the other hand, one study employing psychological tests concluded that in chronic amphetamine users, there was no evidence to support the contention that the drug contributes directly to sexual disturbance (Greaves 1972).

Diethylpropion has also been shown to cause gynaecomastia, and this may result from its effect in releasing luteinizing hormone (Bridgman and Buckler 1974). Mazindol, on the other hand, appears in all the reviews as being aphrodisiac. This follows a single short letter, including one case history (Friesen 1976), citing this as a side effect in 5 per cent of female patients. This incidence was based on a large number of obese patients treated with the drug. In contrast data collected by the manufacturer, both in the UK and world-wide, is quite incompatible with this 'aphrodisiac' report (personal communication from Wander Pharmaceuticals). In a recent 8-year period, there were 16 spontaneous reports of a decrease in libido with this drug, as compared with three reports of an increase. There were additionally 12 cases of 'libido disturbance'. World-wide reports would suggest an incidence of sexual disturbance of 0.06 per cent.

Fenfluramine clearly *decreases* libido in women, this being particularly marked at high doses, with an incidence as high as 85 per cent (Pinder, Brogden, Sawyer, Speight, and Avery 1975). This is compatible with the alleged differences between the sympathomimetics. A role for 5-hydroxytryptamine in sexual enthusiasm has long been advanced (see Chapter 3). Its depletion by *p*-chlorophenylalanine leads to sexual activity, and so its release could decrease libido.

I have dwelt on the sympathomimetic anorectic agents for a disproportionate length because they well illustrate all the problems of this topic outlined earlier. By way of conclusion it is worth pointing out that sexual interest may well increase during and after improvement of body image whilst dieting.

Monoamine oxidase inhibitors

A difference appears to exist between the hydrazine (irreversible) inhibitors (e.g. phenelzine), and the reversible inhibitors (e.g. tranylcypromine). Phenelzine has been reported to cause ejaculatory failure in men and orgasmic failure in women (Blackwell 1981). That this is associated with its hydrazine nature is implied by a similar observation for iproniazid, but not for tranylcypromine, which is puzzling. There are several theoretical ways in which monoamine oxidase inhibitors (MAOIs) could disturb sexual function, e.g. by potentiating catecholamines and 5-hydroxytryptamine, they could interfere with prolactin release (see later). Their mood-elevating activity could also contribute. Why tranylcypromine should lack such activity is difficult to explain, especially since it retains many of the pharmacological characteristics of amphetamine, to which it is clearly related in structure.

Tricyclic and other antidepressants

The fact that tricyclic antidepressants can cause impotence is better known for its irony than for its frequency. The incidence is low, about 0.5–2 per cent (Beaumont 1973). The possible mechanism is interesting. Most texts ascribe the failure of erection to parasympathetic blockade, another accompaniment of the familiar symptoms of dry mouth etc. However, impotence is not a well-documented side effect of atropine. Some circumstances in which atropine-like drugs are used do not lend themselves to exposing sexual side-effects (e.g. anaesthetic premedication, parkinsonism), but elsewhere they have been widely used in gastrointestinal conditions and in motion sickness. Amongst 'atropine-like' drugs, only disopyramide appears in the literature as causing an isolated case of impotence (McHaffie, Guz, and Johnston, 1977). Penile erection following nerve stimulation is clearly classified as being 'atropine resistant' (Bowman and Rand 1980).

Whilst not dismissing this peripheral component to what is an infrequent side effect, the possibility of its mediation via a different mechanism is important. The classical tricyclic antidepressants interfere with various peripheral neuro-transmitters *in vitro*. At low concentration they inhibit noradrenaline uptake (the action historically associated with antidepressant activity) and they antagonise histamine. At slightly higher concentrations acetylcholine is antagonized, but antagonism at α-adrenoceptors also occurs. At higher concentrations there is interference with 5-hydroxytryptamine receptors and uptake, whilst there is also the possibility of dopamine antagonism in the brain. Dopamine and α-adrenoceptor antagonism are often associated, and so there is potential for many other mechanisms of disturbing sexual function.

Antidepressant drugs with profiles of neurochemical action significantly different from this have been developed. They differ in their relative abilities to inhibit the uptake of noradrenaline, dopamine, and of 5-hydroxytryptamine. Sedative action also differs. For example, amitryptyline is far more sedative than the others and sedation *per se* will confuse interpretation of sexual dysfunction. Most importantly there are differences in the extent of atropine-like activity, and, as is well known, the newer drugs such as mianserin and nomifensin, have less activity than the older ones. Only time will tell whether impotence is less likely to occur with these derivatives, thereby providing evidence for this mechanism of impotence one way or the other.

Lithium salts

Following a chequered introduction into psychiatry, salts of lithium maintain a unique place in therapy; not a common pharmacological property. The incidence of sexual dysfunction attributed to lithium is rare. A few cases of a reduction in sexual interest, without impairment of subsequent performance, have been reported (Lorimy, Lôo, and Deniker 1977), whilst reversible erectile difficulty has been described elsewhere (Vinarová, Uhlíř, Stika, and Vinar 1972).

Whilst not necessarily suggesting that these slightly conflicting reports might reflect differences in ethnic idiosyncrasy, it does seem an interesting additional complication to the interpretation of reports of sexual dysfunction.

Lithium ions facilitate noradrenaline uptake and decrease noradrenaline release, whilst 5-hydroxytryptamine is not affected in a similar way, and this may be important. This decreased noradrenergic activity both centrally and peripherally, could be the cause of sexual disturbance, but it is stressed that the side effect is rare. In addition the drug has a low therapeutic index. It interferes with some hormone functions (notably thyroid), and concurrently taken drugs may aggravate sexual side effects; notably diuretics, antipsychotic and anxiolytic drugs.

Neuroleptics

Our greatest understanding of the mechanism of drug-induced sexual dysfunction centres around prolactin and the drugs that interfere with it. Flückiger (1982) has recently reviewed the mechanisms by which prolactin release can be increased or inhibited.

Most attention has been concentrated on the inhibitory action of dopamine and the consequent releasing action of dopamine antagonists, but many other neurotransmitters may be involved. Both γ-aminobutyric acid and, more importantly, acetylcholine can also inhibit release, thereby providing other targets of drug action. Acetylcholine seems to be the forgotten transmitter in the brain. The opiates, including the endorphins, release prolactin, thereby providing a mechanism for the well documented endocrinological changes that occur during opiate dependence (Mirin, Meyer, Mendelson and Ellingboe 1980). This release of prolactin is probably mediated via dopamine pathways (Kosterlitz 1980).

The endorphins have been suggested as having a role in orgasm in view of the orgasmic nature of diamorphine-induced euphoria, though Goldstein's classic paper implies a lack of effect of naloxone on the course of orgasm in a male volunteer (Goldstein and Hansteen 1977). However an involvement of endorphins in the emotional component of orgasm is still attractive, and Riley has found a dose-related reduction in 'satisfaction' (defined as a relief from sexual tension) following relatively low doses of naloxone (personal communication). Histamine has also been associated with prolactin release mechanisms, and this may contribute to the impotence reported following use of the H_2-receptor antagonist cimetidine, though this drug's anti-androgenic activity could contribute (Millar 1979). Whilst this aspect is beyond the scope of this review, numerous psychoactive drugs possess antihistaminic activity, and this further confuses the picture.

Mechanisms controlling the release of luteinizing hormone remain another target for drug action, and this possible effect of catecholamines was alluded to earlier. Luteinizing hormone release causes increased synthesis of both testosterone and oestrogens, thereby disturbing their normal balance, with resultant gynaecomastia. The dopamine antagonists release prolactin, and impotence is well documented and not infrequent; a figure of 60 per cent for thioridazine was mentioned earlier. In that same report the incidence of sexual dysfunction with other neuroleptics was 25 per cent. In women thioridazine has been reported to reduce the satisfaction of orgasm and cause amenorrhoea. Whilst dopamine antagonism is important, other actions may be involved. Chlorpromazine is a more effective antagonist at α-adrenoceptors than at dopamine receptors, thereby providing a second cause of dysfunction, in this case in the periphery, by inhibiting sympathetic mediated ejaculation. Note also the dry orgasm that can occur due to inadequate closure of the bladder neck with retrograde emission (Kotin *et al* 1976). Further, α-adrenoceptor blockade would seem to be the mechanism of action in some rare cases of drug induced priapism caused by the phenothiazines, including chlorpromazine (Meiraz and Fishelovitch 1969) and thioridazine (Dorman and Schmidt 1976). Since α-blockers are so rarely used *per se*, the condition is very rare, though support for a causal relationship is derived from the observation that labetolol, which has both α- and β-adrenoceptor activity, has also been reported to delay detumescence (Riley, Riley, and Davies 1982) and cause priapism (Law, Copeland, Armistead, and Gabriel 1980).

BETA−ADRENOCEPTOR ANTAGONISTS

The β-blockers are now used quite extensively in psychiatry and even more extensively outside it. It well illustrates one of the problems in this field, that although the β-blockers have been in use for almost 20 years, it was not until 1976 that they were described as a possible cause of impotence (Knarr 1976), which is now a recognized side effect of these compounds.

In a study of 46 male patients, 15 per cent had failure of erection, and in a further 28 per cent there was impairment of erection (Burnett and Chahine 1979). These are high proportions. Dose dependency was shown in this study and this is of importance in view of the high doses used in psychiatry. Impotence during antihypertensive therapy is well known, and there are clearly differences in mechanism of action in relation to different drugs, as, for example, the failure of ejaculation caused by the adrenergic neurone blocking drugs. It is difficult to see in this instance why β-blockade should cause impotence. Some have suggested that an α-receptor dominance becomes exaggerated during β-blockade, causing vasoconstriction (Forsberg, Gustavii, Höjerback and Olsson 1979). However, a central mechanism cannot be ruled out (Knarr 1976; Bathen 1978), although that is what pharmacologists tend to claim when they do not understand the nature of the mechanism involved. On the other hand there is currently intense research on central actions of β-blockers, especially their interaction with tryptaminergic mechanisms (e.g. Turner 1979).

Drug–disease interactions

Two further points are worth making. The trial quoted in the preceding paragraph (Burnett and Chahine 1979), may be a little suspect because it is unclear what other medication the patients were taking. It is likely that they were also taking diuretics which at that time were not considered to be associated with impotence, but are now known to share this side effect (Peart, Barnes, Broughton,

Dollery, Green, Greenberg, Hudson, Lever, Meade, Rose, and Miall 1981). Secondly, impotence caused by antihypertensives must always be assessed against the higher incidence of impotence in hypertensive patients. In untreated hypertensives, the proportion of impotence was found to be 17 per cent compared with a control population of 7 per cent (Griffin 1981). Nevertheless, there does seem to be an association between β-blockers and impotence, and at least five other β-blockers have been mentioned in this context.

Interestingly there are at least two reports of sexual function being restored on changing to a different β-blocker (Bathen 1978; Riley 1980), and both authors stress that the replacement drug does not cross the blood–brain barrier. Perhaps the conclusion of Robinson (1978) that impotence attributable to β-blockers is rare, is numerically nearer the mark, and may perhaps equally apply to *any* antihypertensive agent irrespective of mechanism of action. A second type of dysfunction associated with β-blockers, namely Peyronie's disease, is worth mentioning since, though unusual, it is particularly distressing for the patient. β-blockers have again been implicated, though a causal relationship cannot be established because the disorder occurs more frequently where there is atherosclerosis or indeed hypertension itself (Laake 1981).

CENTRAL DEPRESSANTS

These comprise anxiolytics, sedatives, and hypnotics, the major differences between them being in relation to dose. Impotence with or without a change in libido following sedatives is well known, and some are alleged to decrease libido. There must be at least some other readers who have attempted to release bromine from NAAFI tea! That most famous of anxiolytics, ethanol, has a legendary effect on both libido and subsequent performance that has been the source of many aphorisms, describing the condition, some less subtle than others. Even Shakespeare had a word for it.

The benzodiazepines

Away from licensed premises, the most numerous central depressants consumed are those related to the benzodiazepines. Since the mid-1960s there has been a steady increase in the prescribing of these drugs, to a current figure of about 25 million prescriptions from general practitioners in England alone. Diazepam is now the most commonly prescribed of any drug in the UK. Between 10 and 20 per cent of the adult population of the UK are taking benzodiazepines, and in a clinic dealing with sexual problems the figure is nearer 70 per cent.

It is quite clear that these drugs do not cause impotence. In 1964 Hughes reported a single case of ejaculatory failure associated with chlordiazepoxide, which was reversible on drug discontinuation. Since then chlordiazepoxide has appeared in every review as a cause of impotence, alongside thioridazine and other neuroleptics. Hughes (1982, personal communication) has not seen a similar case since. By a rough calculation, since that time there have been between 250 and 300 million prescriptions for benzodiazepines dispensed from pharmacies in England alone. If prescribing worldwide is considered, it becomes clear that this is the rarest drug side effect. The situation may become different with the ever increasing problem of benzodiazepine dependence, but Lader does not consider it a problem now (personal communication). As far as sexual response is concerned, it seems quite clear that if taken in excess benzodiazepines will decrease it, as will any other sedative.

All the recent work on the benzodiazepine receptors, the link with GABA and its proliferating receptors and the possibility of an endogenous ligand, does not detract from the fact that the progressive depression of the central nervous system caused by increasing intoxication by diazepam, is qualitatively similar to that following ethanol. The apparent lack of effect of these drugs on say, orgasm, is probably due to the circumstance of their taking rather than to any major pharmacological difference.

CONCLUSIONS

A final point concerns the incidence of drug-induced sexual dysfunction. When a drug is introduced on to the market, its side effects are claimed to be basically zero, but after a while side effects become apparent and they attract much publicity. Interest in the drug falls. After a longer time, careful studies are evaluated and the drug establishes its place in the formulary, its therapeutic effects are balanced against its side effects. Examples of drug-induced sexual dysfunction are recorded at different points on this biphasic pattern.

Cooper (1972) has listed all organic causes of impotence, including anatomical, cardiovascular, pharmacological, endocrinological, haematological, infectious, and neurological causes. This is a vast range of mechanisms. In this short review consideration has only been given to a limited number of drugs given in certain circumstances. Sexual dysfunction caused by hormones, cytotoxic, and antihypertensive drugs has not been considered, nor has the considerable problem of drug abuse been discussed. Nevertheless, Cooper stresses that all these organic causes of impotence put together, contribute to less than 5 per cent of all cases of impotence, psychogenic factors being infinitely more important.

References

Bathen, J. (1978). Propranolol erectile dysfunction relieved. *Ann. Int. Med.* **88**, 716–17.
Beaumont, G. (1973). Sexual side effects of clomipramine. *J. Int. Med. Res.* **1**, 469–72.
Blackwell, B. (1981). Antidepressant drugs. In *Side effects of drugs annual* (ed. M. N. G. Dukes) pp. 19–20. Excerpta Medica, Amsterdam.
Bowman, W. C. and Rand, M. J. (1980). In *Textbook of pharmacology*, 2nd Ed., p. 10.13. Blackwell, Oxford.
Bridgman, J. F. and Buckler, J. M. H. (1974). Drug-induced gynaecomastia. *Br. Med. J.*, 24th Aug., 520–1.
Burnett, W. C. and Chahine, R. A. (1979). Sexual dysfunction as a complication of propranolol therapy in man. *Cardiovasc. Med.* **4**, 811–15.
Cooper, A. J. (1972). The causes and management of impotence. *Postgrad. Med. J.* **48**, 548–52.
Couper-Smartt, J. D. and Rodham, R. (1973). A technique for surveying side-effects of tricyclic drugs with reference to reported sexual effects. *J. Int. Med. Res.* **1**, 473–6.

Dorman, B. W. and Schmidt, J. D. (1976). Association of priapism in pheno-thiazine therapy. *J. Urol.* **116**, 51–3.

Flückiger, E. (1982). Inhibitors of prolactin secretion. In *Advances in pharmacology and therapeutics II* (eds. H. Yoshida, Y. Hagihara, and S. Ebashi) Vol. 1, *CNS Pharmacology–Neuropeptides*, pp. 129–44. Pergamon, Oxford.

Forsberg, L., Gustavii, B., Höjerback, T., and Olsson, A. M. (1979). Impotence, smoking and β-blocking drugs. *Fertil. Steril.* **31**, 589–91.

Friesen, L. V. C. (1976). Aphrodisia with mazindol. *Lancet* ii, 974.

Garattini, S. (1980). Recent studies on anorectic agents. *Tr. Pharmac. Sci.* **1**, 354–56.

General Practitioner Research Group (1972). Thioridazine as an antidepressant. *Practitioner* **209**, 95–98.

Goldstein, A. and Hansteen, R. W. (1977). Evidence against involvement of endorphins in sexual arousal and orgasm in man. *Arch. Gen. Psychiat.* **34**, 1179–80.

Greaves, G. (1972). Sexual disturbance among chronic amphetamine users. *J. Nerv. Ment. Dis.* **155**, 363–5.

Griffin, J. P. (1981). Drug-induced sexual dysfunction. In *Iatrogenic diseases*, Update to 2nd Ed, (eds. P. F. d'Arcy and J. P. Griffin) pp. 197–204. Oxford University Press.

Horowitz, J. D. and Goble, A. J. (1979). Drugs and impaired male sexual function. *Drugs* **18**, 206–17.

Hughes, J. M. (1964). Failure to ejaculate with chlordiazepoxide. *Am. J. Psychiat.* **121**, 610–11.

Knarr, J. W. (1976). Impotence from propranolol? *Ann. Int. Med.* **85**, 259.

Kosterlitz, H. W. (1980). Possible physiological roles of the enkephalins and endorphins. In *Clinical pharmacology and therapeutics:* Proceedings of the First World Conference (ed. P. Turner), p. 40. Macmillan, London.

Kotin, J., Wilbert, D. E., Verburg, D., and Soldinger, S. M. (1976). Thioridazine and sexual dysfunction. *Am. J. Psychiat.* **133**, 82–5.

Laake, K. (1981). Anti-anginal and β-adrenoceptor blocking drugs. In *Side effects of drugs annual* (ed. M. N. G. Dukes) p. 187. Excerpta Medica, Amsterdam.

Law, M. R., Copeland, R. F. P., Armistead, J. G., and Gabriel, R. (1980). Labetolol and priapism. *Br. Med. J.*, 12th Jan, 115.

Lorimy, F., Lôo, H., and Deniker, P. (1977). Effets clinique des traitements prolongés par les sels de lithium sur le sommeil, l'appétit et la sexualité. *Encéphale* **3**, 227–39.

McHaffie, D. J., Guz, A., and Johnston, A. (1977). Impotence in patient on disopyramide. *Lancet* i, 859.

Millar, J. G. B. (1979). Drug induced impotence. *Practitioner* **233**, 634–9.

Meiraz, D. and Fishelovitch, J. (1969). Priapism and Largactil medication. *Isr. J. Med. Sci.* **5**, 1254.

Mirin, S. M., Meyer, R. E., Mendelson, J. H. and Ellingboe, J. (1980). Opiate use and sexual function. *Am. J. Psychiat.* **137**, 909–15.

Peart, W. S., Barnes, G. R., Broughton, P., Dollery, C. T., Green, K. G., Greenberg, G., Hudson, M. F., Lever, A. F., Meade, T. W., Rose, G. A., and Miall, W. E. (1981). Adverse reactions to bendrofluazide and propranolol for the treatment of mild hypertension. *Lancet* ii 539–43.

Pinder, R. M., Brogden, R. N., Sawyer, P. R., Speight, T. M. and Avery, G. S. (1975). Fenfluramine: a review of its pharmacological properties and therapeutic efficacy in obesity. *Drugs* **10**, 241–323.

Riley, A. J. (1980). Antihypertensive therapy and sexual function. *Br. J. Sex. Med.* **7**, 23–7.

Riley, A. J., Riley, E. J., and Davies, H. J. (1982). A method for monitoring drug effects on male sexual reponse: the effect of single dose labetolol. *Br. J. Clin. Pharmac.* **14**, 695–700.

Robinson, B. F. (1978). Anti-anginal and β-adrenoceptor blocking drugs. In *Side effects of drugs annual* (ed. M. N. G. Dukes), p. 170. Excerpta Medica, Amsterdam.

Seagraves, R. T. (1979). Sexual dysfunction and psychotropic drugs. *Br. J. Sex. Med.* **6**, 51–2.

Tolley, P. H. and Lack, C. (1949). Gynaecomastia during treatment with amphetamine. *Lancet* **i**, 650–1.

Turner, P. (1979). Central nervous actions of β-adrenoceptor blocking drugs in man. *Tr. Pharmac. Sci.* **1**, 49–51.

Vinařová, E., Uhliř, O., Stika, L., and Vinar, O. (1972). Side effects of lithium administration. *Act. Nerv. Super. (Praha).* **14**, 105–7.

Wheatley, D. (1972). Thioridazine and impotence. *Practitioner,* **209**, 585–6.

12

Aphrodisiacs – in legend and in fact

ROBERT B. GREENBLATT, CHRISTIAN VERHEUGEN,
JASWANT CHADDHA, AND CONSTANTINE SAMARAS

INTRODUCTION

Modern man and woman are throwing off the shackles of sexual repression.
The adolescent is in revolt, whilst more mature individuals are wondering if
they have taken advantage of their inherent gifts for sexual gratification and,
if failing to achieve sexual fulfilment, why nature and circumstance have passed
them by. The ageing couple wonder if their lovemaking days need draw to a
close.

In dealing so unabashedly with sexuality, the mass media have stirred up
a hornet's nest, unloosing inhibitions, stirring fantasies, destroying cherished
traditions and taboos, and creating an urgency for sexual experimentation.
We find ourselves in the throes of a sexual revolution: changing values, greater
permissiveness, a new morality. Detaching sex from love has meant sexual
evolution for some, sexual revulsion for others. An enlightened society, indeed
an aroused one, thirsts for knowledge, whilst advice, both good and bad, appears
in medical journals, lay magazines, and an assortment of books. The psychiatrist,
marriage counsellor, clergyman, and physician are expected to show expertise
in this highly complicated field.

THE ROLE OF APHRODISIACS

Sexual behaviour is the sum total of the individual makeup, including chromosomal sex, gender identification, gonadal adequacy, childhood rearing, environmental influences, possible hypothalamic sensitization, and hormonal factors.
Much has been written about the importance of the psyche in matters of sex,
and of the mechanics of coitus as well as the proper amatory prelude. The time
is ripe for an assessment as to whether aphrodisiacs, past or present, modify
sexual responsiveness, but more importantly to dispel the notion current in
many circles that hormonal therapy is of little value. Human endocrinopathies
have aided the endocrinologist to delineate the role of gonads, chromosomal
endowment, socio-environmental factors, exogenous and endogenous hormones,
not only in sexual development but also in psycho-sexual orientation and
gender identity. We can approach the problems of sexual adjustment more
easily if we can understand the part played by the psyche and that of the endo-
crines in sexual behaviour.

Some 40 years ago, when writing about sexual matters was not in vogue, one
of us (R.B.G.) stated that libido was a chemical test-tube equation. Although

neurological, psychogenic, anatomical, pathological, and nutritional factors play important roles, the essential hormone for positive sex drive in both male and female is testosterone (Greenblatt, Montara, and Torpin 1942). Time and experience involving thousands of patients have fortified this posture. We realize the complexity of sex and readily acknowledge that the 'test-tube equation' concept is an oversimplification. It is paramount that we appreciate the fact that considerable numbers of men and women are in need of help; relatively few can avail themselves of the benefits offered by the few centres for sexual study, or a prolonged course of psychoanalysis.

Since early antiquity, human beings have sought ways by which sexual desire could be stimulated or intensified. Drugs or food which seemed effective were appropriately named after Aphrodite, the goddess of love and beauty in Greek mythology, and 'aphrodisiacs' have always been of interest to mankind. Aphrodisiacal properties have been attributed to certain foods, herbs, plants, alcoholic beverages, powdered Rhinoceros horn, and specific drugs. Save for testosterone, and that too has been questioned, no pharmacological agent or any plant or foodstuff, has yet been found which directly increases sexual capacity and performance. If effectiveness has been claimed, the power of suggestion has been grossly underestimated. There are eager people throughout the world who will pay any price for an aphrodisiac, forgetting that the last he or she bought or concocted, had no effect or at best a fleeting one. Some of the love potions or philtres used in the past and present merit comment.

Herbs and plants

Mandrake has been touted for centuries as an aphrodisiac, because of the biblical account that Rachel overcame her infertility, after bargaining with Leah for her son Reuben's mandrakes. Perhaps no plant has been more widely praised than this one, and, in fact, the brew of the mandrake was one of the earliest tranquillizers in use. Although Dioscorides, the Greek physician who practised in Rome during the first Century AD, employed the wine of mandragora as an anodyne, he also believed it to have aphrodisiacal powers. The mandrake (*Mandragora officinarum*), a plant growing wild in the Mid-East, often miscalled the May apple or Devil's apple, is the source of more superstitions than any other plant. Its long and twisted root roughly resembles the human form, and it has been credited with many properties: to bring sleep, to kill pain, to increase wealth, to arouse ardour, and to overcome barrenness. The 'Song' of John Donne (1573–1631), Dean of St. Paul's, plays on this belief:

> goe, and catche a falling starre,
> get with child a mandrake roote.

The roots of the orchid sometimes resemble testicles (orchid from the greek word meaning gonad), and because of this, orchid roots were believed to be sexual stimulants. One kind much sought after was known as Satyrion (after the lecherous satyrs) and another, 'autumn lady's tresses', was sometimes referred to as sweet cullion (Chaucer used the word cullion for testicle). These, when eaten or boiled in milk and drunk, were said to 'provoke venery'. Women of

Thesaly made a potion of tubers of certain orchids to excite desire and tubers are still gathered in many parts of Europe and Asia for such purposes. Legend has it that Hercules drank a beverage of tubers dissolved in goats milk which so kindled the fires of desire that he deflowered 50 virgins in one night.

Lost in antiquity are many herbs that were used as aphrodisiacs, and one of these was called 'Moly'. Homer spoke of the powers of this herb to excite passion, whilst Milton wrote: '. . . moly that Hermes to wise Ulysses gave', and Tennyson of: '. . . beds of amaranth and moly.'

Alcoholic beverages

Neolithic man, turning from hunting to agriculture, soon learned to use his crops for fermentation. People in various parts of the Earth found that grapes or wet grain, allowed to stand in warmth, became a liquor which possessed weird and pleasant effects. The world's first biochemists probably were those primitive people who concerned themselves with the fermentation of grain for beer and grapes for wine. The earliest reference to wine in the Bible points out that excessive intake leads to lewdness and inordinate sexual behaviour. 'And Noah began to be a husbandman, and he planted a vineyard: And he drank of the wine and was drunken; and he was uncovered within his tent' (Genesis 9: 20–21). The much embarrassed sons of Noah 'covered their father's nakedness'. Wine and alcoholic beverages have been used at all times and in all climes to remove inhibitions and promote sexuality, but Shakespeare aptly warned, 'and drink, sir, is a great provoker . . . it provokes the desire, but it takes away the performance', (Macbeth II, 3).

Foodstuffs

The word honeymoon is derived from the old North European custom of drinking honeyed wine or mead to promote sexual desires during the first month of marriage. Honey is still esteemed by many as an aphrodisiac. Hippocrates thought so and on his advice cakes made from asses milk and honey were eaten as a food of love. In the sixteenth century the French mistakenly presumed that the tomato was an aphrodisiac and gave to this fruit the name 'pomme d'amour' − love apple. In England love apples were frowned upon as being conducive to excessive passion.

Oysters, octopus, and red mullet have been favoured as aphrodisiacs, and to this day sea-food lovers believe them to be supportive of sexual powers. Another claimed aphrodisiac, powdered rhinoceros horn, is in insatiable demand in India and the Far East. There are those who firmly believe that this organic material directly influences sexual performance and erectile capacity.

PSYCHODYNAMIC PROCEDURES

Pornography

The description of explicit sexual acts and sexual imagery often proves stimulating and intriguing to those in search of some mechanism that might trigger a surge in their sexual drive. The Song of Solomon was nearly excluded from the

Holy Bible because the pious considered the imagery lewd and pagan. The Reverend E. P. Eddruff, Prebendary of Salisbury Cathedral, admonished that such a book as The Song of Solomon, may not be fitted for public reading in a mixed congregation or even in private by the pure of heart (Greenblatt 1963). Pornography is an evaluative term, often used pejoratively to designate explicit material deliberately designed to stimulate sexual arousal and sexual fantasies. Voyeurism could certainly be included under the broad heading of pornography.

Flagellation

Assaulting areas of the body close to the genitals by whips and chains causes a rush of blood to the area and this, it has been reported, is followed quickly by intense desire. The psychogenic aspects of this form of flagellation were appreciated by the Marquis de Sade, who wrote on the relationship between pain and sexual gratification.

Power

Kissinger is alleged to have said that power is the greatest aphrodisiac. Fame and fortune nurture greater liberties and dimensions in sexual comportment, and accounts of the bizarre sexual activities of famous and infamous people who have influenced the tides of history, are legion. The struggle for dominance, it appears, is linked with excessive sexual drive which increases dramatically with success, and the power-sex syndrome consumes many leaders whom the world either reveres or hates. Kings, queens, statesmen, dictators, and politicians often display relentless sexual urges, normal or deviant, to match their power, fame, and exalted positions. There has always been one set of rules for the mighty and the rich, another for the common man. Did not Mussolini shut down the brothel house of Rome, yet hardly a day passed without him seducing one or more women? His devoted mistress Claretta Petacci once exclaimed wrathfully to a friend, 'he has these women seven at a time' (Greenblatt 1978).

PHARMACEUTICAL AGENTS

Cantharides

Cantharides is an alleged aphrodisiac which has enjoyed popular usage for the past few centuries. Glamorous mystery surrounds the preparation of 'Spanish Fly' from dried beetles, especially blister beetles. Cantharides is toxic to the genito-urinary tract producing bladder irritation, urinary frequency, and occasionally priapism. Although highly esteemed as an aphrodisiac it has proved worthless. In his play *Les Deux Biscuits*, Grandval, in 1715, referred to Spanish Fly:

> L'un était composé de mouche cantharides
> Qui redonnent la force aux amants invalides.

Yohimbine

For many years yohimbine has been considered to be an aphrodisiac. Many biologists have long believed that the bark of the yohimbee tree contained a pharmacological agent that had physiological activity capable of alleviating erectile dysfunction. Recently numerous studies have clarified some of its pharmacological properties. It is an α-adrenolytic agent, that selectively enhances the release of noradrenaline (norepinephrine) by nerve endings. Morales, Surridge, and Marshall (1981) of Queens University, Canada, in giving 6 mg three times daily to six diabetics with organic erectile failure, obtained improvement in four for as long as medication was continued. A decrease in the noradrenaline content of the corpus cavernosum has been documented in diabetics with erectile failure (Levine 1976).

Marijuana

In a study performed on 100 regular marijuana users in order to determine the order of side effects, Halikas, Goodwin, and Guze (1971) found that one third of the group noted a greater than 50 per cent degree of sexual arousal and improvement of sexual performance.

Steroid hormones

Hormonal interactions with catechols in the 5-hydroxytryptamine chain, such as serotonin and other neurotransmitters, may be instrumental in the modification of sexual behaviour (Zitrin, Dement, Barchas *et al.* 1973). Alterations in the ratio of dopamine to serotonin in the brain can markedly affect sexual function in male rats (Gessa and Tagliamonte 1975). The aphrodisiac effects of neurotransmitter manipulation were first suggested by O'Malley (1981), when he noticed that some male patients exhibited heightened sexual interest while taking L-dopa in the treatment of parkinsonism. L-Dopa, which is the immediate precursor of the neurotransmitter dopamine, acted as a stimulant in about 4–30 per cent of cases, and three times more often in men than women.

It has long been known that sex steroids strongly influence the neurotransmitters of the brain. Sexuality in both males and females depends, in large part, upon the activity of the reproductive hormones. Castration of pre-adolescent males and ovarian extirpation in pre-adolescent females, results in loss of sexual drive. Many examples of the role of steroid hormones in nature's experiments, have yielded significant facts. Women with virilizing adrenal tumours, congenital adrenal hyperplasia, or masculinizing ovarian neoplasms, frequently display sexual aggressiveness, even to the extent of nymphomania (Table 12.1). On the other hand, individuals suffering from hypercortisolism (Cushing's syndrome), hypoadrenalism (Addison's disease), or hyperprolactinaemia, display marked loss in sexual drive. In trials using either androgens or oestrogens in the management of women suffering from advanced mammary cancer, some moribund cachectic women experienced uncontrollable sexual urges while on large doses of testosterone but this did not occur with oestrogens. Furthermore, a careful scrutiny of women on oral contraceptives and on long-acting progestogens reveals that the preliminary effect of freedom from possible unwanted conception, resulted in an increase in sexual gratification. However, with prolonged use, a goodly proportion of women reported gradual loss of sexual drive.

A greater understanding of human endocrinopathies is aiding the physician

TABLE 12.1 *Personality changes and biochemical data – three sisters with congenital adrenal hyperplasia*

Personality disorder	Age (yrs)	Ur. Excretion (mg/24 hrs)		Response to Cortisone	Age at:				Onset of virilization
		17-Keto steroids	Pregnane-triol		Menarche	Cessation of menses	Appearance of pubic hair		
1. Nymphomania with homosexual tendencies*	34	35.9 18.6	24.5	Good	10	18	4		18
2. Religious fanatic	44	75.2	–	Good	11	15	?		15
3. Alcoholic†	51	43.0	23.5	Refused Rx	0	–	9		?

*During cortisone therapy, libido returned to normal and homosexual tendencies disappeared.
†Surgery (abdominal) was performed at age 17. She had not menstruated before operation and did not menstruate afterward. (Possibly the operation was a panhysterectomy). Reproduced from Greenblatt, R. B., and Leng, J. -J. (1972). Factors influencing sexual behavior. *J. Am. Geriatrics* **20**, 49, with permission of the authors.

to delineate the role of hormones in sexual development and in human sexuality. Androgens appear to increase the responsiveness of certain central nervous system mechanisms to peripheral excitation; progestogens, with rare exception, seem to diminish that response. These effects are sometimes clouded by sublimation and modification of the urge for sexual gratification, by learning experience, and culture. The intrusion of psychic factors, however, merely modifies sexual arousal and responsiveness.

SEXUAL BEHAVIOUR IN THE FEMALE

Primarily, sexuality may depend on the state of the endocrine glands, and young women suffering from sexual infantilism are usually completely devoid of sex drive. The cause may be congenital (i.e. primary ovarian failure) or early ovarian failure. Loss of ovarian function can be secondary to a hypothalamic lesion, as occurs in Kallmann's syndrome (hypo-ovarianism with anosmia), because of the absence of luteinizing hormone-releasing factor (LHRF), Lacking LHRF, the pituitary is not stimulated to produce gonadotropins. Secondary ovarian failure may be due either to an inherent inability to manufacture gonadotropins, or to loss of that capacity because of a chromophobe tumour or a craniopharyngioma, which replaces or destroys the pituitary. Other pituitary tumours, such as prolactinomas (amenorrhoea/galactorrhoea syndrome), ACTH-producing tumours (Cushing's disease), and acidophilic cell tumours (acromegaly), also may be associated with loss of sex drive.

Some women experience heightened sex interest at the time of ovulation and others during the week prior to the menstrual period. However, many women find sexual relations during the latter part of the luteal phase less than appealing. Animal experiments indicate similar reactions. The female baboon's sex skin is red during the peak of the follicular phase, a visual sign of sexual preparedness; it blanches during the luteal phase when the female fights off male advances.

Influence of dyspareunia

Dyspareunia causes interest in sex to wane in oestrogen-deficient women because of atrophy of the vaginal mucosa, and the use of oestrogens (oral, parenteral, topical) may suffice to overcome dyspareunia. Many clinicians add a small amount of androgen to an oestrogen regimen, because it contributes to the woman's sense of well-being and rekindles waning sex drive. Menopausal women desire sexual fulfilment just as younger women do and adequate hormone replacement therapy facilitates the attainment of these hopes. On the other hand, many women at menopause, freed from the fear of pregnancy, experience an increase in sex drive, which may be excessive in some.

Dyspareunia and avoidance of sexual relations may occur in women suffering from endometriosis. The use of danazol, progestational agents, and/or testosterone may afford temporary relief. Kraurosis vulvae, a moderately rare but advanced form of atrophic vulvitis and vaginitis, is complicated by regressive changes in the perigenital skin, narrowing of the vaginal introitus, and unrelenting pruritus. The local use of ointments containing hydrocortisone or its analogues, and of oestrogens (oral or parenteral), ameliorates the discomfort, assuages the pruritus, and tends to overcome the incapacity for sex.

Hormone treatment

Sexual dysfunction may be primary or secondary. Primary absence of sexual desire in normally menstruating women is regarded as psychogenic in origin, and frequently requires the efforts of the endocrinologist, psychiatrist, and a competent team of sex counsellors. Women who previously had sexual drive, but lost it, usually are far easier to manage. Reduced libido is often seen in a woman who has had many pregnancies and is fatigued and bored by the burdens of child care and household chores. The glow of the sexual encounter may have faded, but in most instances her sexual response may be revived readily by the administration of androgenic hormones (Fig. 21.1). Certainly, correction of environmental problems is of the utmost importance; but, despite untoward influences, testosterone administration restores the capacity for sexual gratification in about 75 per cent of women who have experienced sexual desire previously. Oestrogens alone are not, or are only occasionally, effective; except in the case of dyspareunia resulting from dryness of the vaginal canal due to oestrogen lack, as in atrophic vaginitis.

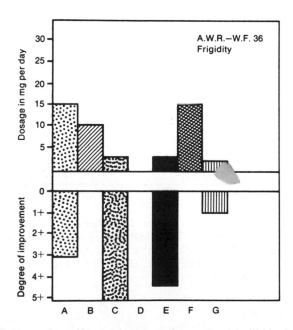

FIG. 12.1 Comparative effects of various hormones on libido in 36-year-old woman complaining of frigidity. Responses (+ to 5+) shown in the lower part; sequence of hormone dosages shown in the upper part, from left to right: A, methyltestosterone; B, placebo; C, testosterone by implantation; D, no therapy; E, testosterone propionate s.c.; F, progestogens; and G, oestrogens. (Reproduced from Greenblatt, R. B. and Leng, J. -J. (1978).

The hormone of libido is testosterone. In the adult female, the administration of androgens does not alter the form of the motor acts involved in courtship and mating; it merely increases susceptibility to sexual excitement. In a double-blind study using an oestrogen, an androgen, and a placebo, it was noted that the combination of oestrogen and androgen, or androgen alone, induced libidinous drives (Table 12.2) (Greenblatt, Barfield, Garner *et al.* 1950). Double-blind studies suggest that androgens profoundly influence sexual behaviour in the female. While oestrogens may heighten sexual interest, and progestogens may dampen sexual desire, it is androgens, in non-virilizing doses, that can restore libidinous drives in the majority of women with sexual dysfunction (Fig. 12.2) (Studd 1978).

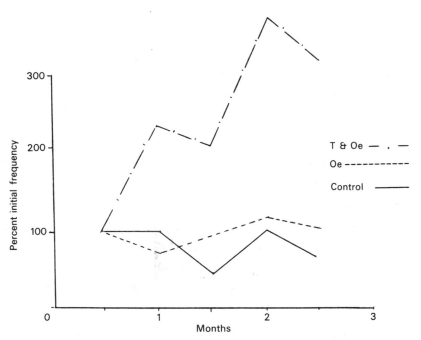

FIG. 12.2. Percentage increase in orgasm following implantation of testosterone 100 mg plus oestradiol 50 mg (T + Oe); oestradiol 30 mg (Oe); and placebo. (Courtesy of Studd, J. W. W. (1979). The climacteric syndrome, in *Female and Male Climacteric* (eds. P. A. van Keep, D. M. Serr, and R. B. Greenblatt) pp. 23–34. MTP Press, Lancaster.

THE MALE PATIENT

The problem of sexual dysfunction in the male is more complex than in the female. In the male particularly, libido refers only to desire for sex, whereas erectile dysfunction or impotence refers to a male's ability to achieve and maintain an erection sufficient for vaginal intromission.

TABLE 12.2 *Double-blind studies: androgens increased libido while oestrogens did so only slightly at times.*

Therapy	Courses of therapy		Percentage of patients				
	Private	Clinic	With nausea	With increased libido	With acne, hoarseness, or hirsutism	With intact uterus and bleeding following treatment	With no improvement
AE-1 Diethylstilbestrol, 0.25 mg	67	21	30.5	12.3	0	34.2	3.1
AE-2 Diethylstilbestrol, 0.25 mg Methyltestosterone, 5.0 mg	54	19	4.0	23.5	13.2	30.5	10.4
AE-3 Methy-testosterone, 5.0 mg	44	19	5.2	42.0	12.8	0.98	23.6
AE-4 Placebo	36	24	3.6	1.8	0	0	83.8

AE: Androgen-oestrogen
Reproduced from Greenblatt *et al.* (1955). *J. Clin. Endocrinol.* **10**, 1547.

Androgens and libido

Several years ago Herrmann and Beach (1976) reviewed the world literature and concluded that there is evidence that androgens have an identifiable impact on certain aspects of behaviour. They referred to it as a 'psychotropic effect'. They found that androgens increase libido in androgen-deficient males, but not in normal males. There is no doubt that testosterone is clearly helpful in hypogonadal men (Davidson, Caimargo, and Smith 1979; Skakkebaek, Bancroft, Davidson, and Warren 1981), whilst there is a subsample of males with erectile dysfunction who can benefit from endocrine therapy. In a group of men with hypogonadism resulting from pituitary tumours, Spark, White and Connolly (1980) restored erectile function in 18 of 19 men with injections of either testosterone enanthate or human chorionic gonadotropin.

Testosterone injections also resulted in a dramatic increase in libido and return of erectile function in castrates and men with hypergonadotropic hypogonadism. They were able also to restore erectile capacity in men suffering from hyperthyroidism when treated with propylthiouracil. Thorner and Besser (1976) restored erectile function with bromocriptine in 19 of 25 patients, 15 of whom had acromegaly, and 5 hyperprolactinaemia. The latter condition is far rarer in men than in women; the administration of testosterone in the presence of hyperprolactinaemia is generally ineffective.

Oral hormone therapy

The percentage of men with endocrinopathies (latent or patent) is relatively low. None the less, many physicians have been wont to administer 5–10 mg doses of oral androgens (methyltestosterone or fluoxymesterone) to all men complaining of erectile dysfunction. Improvement, if any, when it did occur was usually fleeting and probably due to suggestion. Few studies using oral androgens for the treatment of impotence have been well designed or compared with a placebo.

In order to evaluate such oral hormone therapy, our group undertook a double blind study comparing a placebo and methyltestosterone in a group of 20 males, without obvious endocrinopathy, aged 50–78. A 25 mg tablet or a matching placebo tablet was administered daily for 30 days, then increased to two tablets for a further 30 days, then three tablets for a final 30 days. Relatively large doses were used in this 90 day study, because in our experience the usual dosage of 5–10 mg has proved to be no more effective than a placebo. Table 12.3 reveals that there were no excellent responses to the placebo, while there were seven excellent responses on the 25–75 mg trials of methyltestosterone. All in all, the placebo yielded a moderate to good improvement in 12 per cent of the trials; while the hormone yielded moderate, good or excellent in 47 per cent of the trials (Albeaux-Fernet 1978). The potential hepatoxicity of methyltestosterone leading to liver damage and jaundice, together with the risk of side-effects such as gynaecomastia, negate its long term use. In the past, many males with erectile dysfunction have presented in our clinic who had tried Afrodex* (a preparation containing 5 mg nux vomica, 5 mg

TABLE 12.3 *Results of double-blind trial of placebo and methyltestosterone in 20 men (50–78 years of age)*

Dose	No. of trials	Degree of response
Placebo		
1 Tab.	20	+ + in 2
2 Tab.	18	+ + in 2
3 Tab.	17	+ in 1
		+ + in 2
Total	55	7 (12.7%)
Methyltestosterone (25 mg)		
1 Tab.	20	+ in 4
		+ + in 2
		+ + + in 2
2 Tab.	20	+ in 3
		+ + in 4
		+ + + in 2
3 Tab.	19	+ in 3
		+ + in 5
		+ + + in 3
Total	59	28 47.4%

Each trial = 30 days. + = moderate; + + = good; + + + = excellent.
From: Albeaux-Fernet, M., Bohler, C. S-S., and Karpas, A. E. (1978). Testicular function in the aging male. In *Geriatric endocrinology* (ed. R. B. Greenblatt) vol. 5, pp. 201–16. New York, Raven Press.

methyltestosterone and 5 mg yohimbine).* Although we have never employed this poly-pharmaceutical agent, the impression gained from these patients was not impressive.

Effects of age

How about the management of the male 50 years of age and older, who presents with loss of potentia, depression, and irritability or insomnia, after presumably having enjoyed a normal sex life? Is he suffering from environmental influences that are coincidental to his age or is there a hormonal correlation? Generally speaking, FSH and LH levels in the average male aged 50–60 years, either remain within normal limits (8 ± 4 mIU/ml) or increase up to twofold, as compared to postmenopausal females in whom there is an increase of as much as 14 times more FSH and eight times more LH. When men reach the age of 70–80 years, gonadotropin levels begin to approximate those seen in the female menopause and in men with primary testicular failure or following castration (Fig. 12.3). Testosterone levels begin to fall in most males after the age of 50 (Fig. 12.4), especially those with loss of potentia. Relatively small doses of an oral androgen (5–10 mg of methyltestosterone or fluoxymesterone) given to males produce little change in FSH and LH levels. To achieve a marked fall in LH and FSH values, large doses of testosterone are administered either by injection (100 mg depotestosterone cypionate/week) or by implanting

*Not available in Great Britain – Ed.

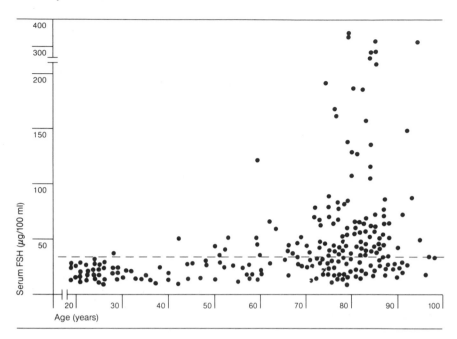

FIG. 12.3   Serum FSH levels in men, 18–97 years of age. Dotted line indicates the upper limit of normal for men less than 45 years of age. (From Stearns, E., MacDonnell, J. A., Kaufman, B. J. *et al.* (1974). Declining testicular function with age: Hormonal and clinical correlates. *Am. J. Med.* **57**, 761.)

submuscularly 10–15 pellets of testosterone into the buttock (Fig. 12.5).

In our clinic, we employ oral androgens but sparingly (methyltestosterone or fluoxymesterone), because more consistent results are obtained with injectables, such as 100 mg of testosterone cypionate at 7–10-day intervals, or by subcutaneous implantation of testosterone pellets (75 mg each), one per 5–10 kg of body weight (Figs. 12.6 and 12.7).

A male with andropausal symptoms is often accused of having psychogenic problems. Many males do have symptoms as a result of low androgen levels, especially when complicated by stress and unfavourable environmental conditions. Symptoms such as depression, headache, and impotence are common complaints. Many of these patients, when given testosterone in adequate amounts, claim improvement in their libidinous drive, capacity for sexual relations, and amelioration of headaches and depression.

CONCLUSIONS

Over the centuries, the means employed to stimulate or revive sexual powers have varied from prayer, magic, herbs, and plants, to methods that might stimulate the sensory organs of sight, hearing, touch, taste, and smell. Best known in Western culture are alcohol, oysters, cantharides, yohimbine, and pornography. With the advent of modern endocrinology, testosterone properly and selectively used has proved to be the only true aphrodisiac. Correction of certain endocrinopathies (antithyroid drugs in hyperthyroidism, bromocriptine in hyper-

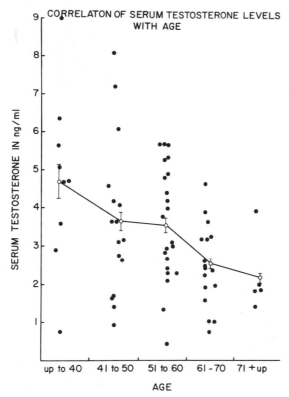

FIG. 12.4 Serum testosterone levels obtained in men with erectile dysfunction. Normal serum testosterone levels > 4 ng/ml.

prolactinaemia) brings endogenous testosterone into balance. There is no doubt that testosterone is effective in hypogonadism; it is also helpful in many sexually dysfunctional males with and without low serum testosterone values, by improving well being and lessening depression. Testosterone, in non-virilizing doses, will, in most instances, increase libido in women who once knew it.

Androgens appear to increase responsiveness of certain central nervous system mechanisms to peripheral excitation. They probably act by way of neurotransmitters and the nervous system; in a measure testosterone is a psychotropic drug.

References

Albeaux-Fernet, M., Bohler, C. S-S., and Karpas, A. E. (1978). Testicular function in the aging male. In *Geriatric endocrinology* (ed. R. B. Greenblatt) pp. 201–16. Raven Press, New York.

Davidson, J., Caimargo, C., and Smith, E. (1979). Effects of androgen on sexual behavior in hypogonadal men. *J. Clin. Endocrinol. Metab.* **48**, 955–8.

Gessa, G. L. and Tagliamonte, A. (1975). Role of brain serotonin and dopamine in male sexual behavior. In *Sexual behavior – pharmacology and biochemistry* (eds. M. Sandler and G. L. Gessa) Raven Press, New York.

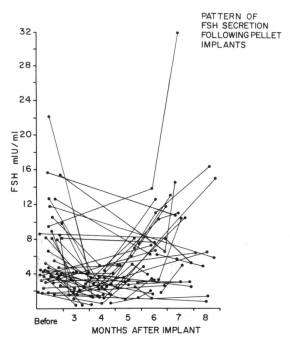

FIG. 12.5 Pattern of FSH secretion following pellet implants. Note fall in FSH values after pellet implantation and gradual return to previous levels as pellets are absorbed.

Greenblatt, R. B. (1963). *Search the Scriptures. Modern medicine and biblical personages.* Lippincott, Philadelphia.
— (1978). *Love lives of the famous — a physician's reflections.* MPT Press, Lancaster.
— Mortara, F., and Torpin, R. (1942). Sexual libido in the female. *Am. J. Obstet. Gynecol.* **44**, 658–63.
— Barfield, W. E., and Garner, J. K. (1950). Evaluation of an estrogen, androgen, estrogen–androgen combination and a placebo in the treatment of the menopause. *J. Clin. Endocrinol.* **10**, 1547–58.
— Oettinger, M. and Bohler, C. S-S. (1976). Estrogen–androgen levels in aging men and women: therapeutic considerations. *J. Am. Geriatr. Soc.* **24**, 173–8.
— Nezhat, C., Roesel, R. A., and Natrajan, P. K. (1979). Update on the male and female climacteric. *J. Am. Geriatr. Soc.* **27**, 481–90.
Halikas, J. A., Goodwin, P. H., and Guze, S. B. (1971). Marijuana effects: a survey of regular users. *JAMA* **217**, 692–4.
Herrmann, W. M. and Beach, R. C. (1976). Psychotropic effects of androgens: a review of clinical observations and new human experimental findings. *Pharmakopsychiatr. Neuropsychopharmakol.* **9**, 205–19.
Levine, S. B. (1976). Marital sexual dysfunction: erectile dysfunction. *Ann. Int. Med.* **85**, 342–50.
Morales, A., Surridge, D. M., and Marshall, P. G. (1981). Yohimbine for treatment of impotence in diabetes. *N. Engl. J. Med.* **305**, 1221.
O'Malley, W. E. (1981). Drugs to boost sexual potency. *Geriatrics* **37**, 158–66.

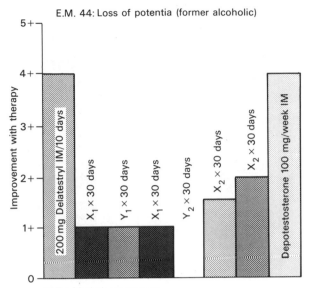

FIG. 12.6   Results following use of methyltestosterone, placebo, and parenteral androgens.

Skakkebaek, N., Bancroft, J., Davidson, D., and Warren, P. (1981). Androgen replacement with oral testosterone undecanoate in hypogonadal men. A double blind controlled study. *Clin. Endocrinol.* **14**, 49–61.

Spark, R., White, R., and Connolly, P. (1980). Impotence is not always psychogenic. *JAMA* **243**, 750–5.

Stearns, E., MacDonnell, J. A., Kaufman, B. J. *et al.* (1974). Declining testicular function with age. Hormonal and clinical correlates. *Am. J. Med.* **57**, 761–6.

Studd, J. W. W. (1978). The climacteric syndrome. In *Female and male climacteric* (eds. P. A. VanKeep, D. M. Serr, and R. B. Greenblatt) pp. 23–33. MTP Press, Lancaster.

Thorner, M. and Besser, G. (1976). Hyperprolactinemia and gonadal function: Results of bromocriptine treatment. In *Serono symposia on prolactin and human reproduction* (eds. P. Crosignani and C. Robyn) Academic Press, New York.

Zitrin, A., Dement, W. C., Barchas, J. D. *et al.* (1973). Brain serotonin and male sexual behavior. In *Contemporary sexual behavior* (eds. J. Zubin and J. Money) pp. 321–36. Johns Hopkins University Press, Baltimore.

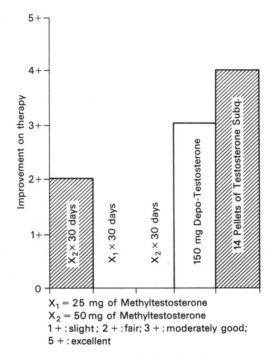

X₁ = 25 mg of Methyltestosterone
X₂ = 50 mg of Methyltestosterone
1 + : slight ; 2 + : fair; 3 + : moderately good;
5 + : excellent

FIG. 12.7 Excellent results following pellet implantation.

13

Drug treatment of hypersexuality

C. J. MUGGLESTONE

INTRODUCTION

The pharmacological management of hypersexuality can be divided for convenience into specific and non-specific treatments. In the specific group we have the anti-androgens, and in the non-specific, the sedatives and neuroleptics. Before considering treatment in further detail, it is useful to consider what is known about the pathogenesis of hypersexuality, and the effects that androgens have on sex-drive and other body functions.

ANDROGENS

The fact that endogenous androgens appear to be necessary for the male sex-drive has been well known for many hundreds of years – without the benefit of radio-immune assays. The Caliphs of Bagdad and the Emperors of China, with their eunuchs to look after the harems, were certainly aware of this and of the major site of their production. More recently Rada, Laws, and Kellner (1976) showed that a group of particularly violent rapists had significantly higher testosterone levels than normal, although other male sex offenders in the same study had normal levels.

Effects in the female

It is only recently that the female sex-drive has also been shown to be affected by androgens. It has been reported that adrenalectomy, which removes the main source of androgens in the female, is followed by a reduction of sexual arousal. Vermeulen and Verdonck (1976) demonstrated that there is a mid-cycle peak of testosterone coinciding with ovulation, which provides a neat physiological mechanism whereby increased sexual receptivity and activity are induced, when fertility is greater.

Although exogenous androgens have been thought for 50 years to enhance sexual responsiveness in the female, it was not until 1978 that Carney, Bancroft, and Mathews demonstrated this in a controlled trial. They compared testosterone to diazepam, with concurrent counselling, in 32 couples complaining of female unresponsiveness, and demonstrated significant increases in the sexual ratings of the testosterone group including:

Pleasant feelings during sexual contact.
Frequency of sexually exciting thoughts.
Frequency of arousal.
Frequency of sexual attractiveness of the male partner.

Frequency of satisfaction with intercourse.

Frequency of orgasm.

The opposite effects have been noted from treatment with anti-androgens. Similarly, oestrogens which are known to increase sex hormone binding globulin (SHBG), thereby reducing free testosterone, also decrease sexual drive in the male. It is established that androgens are essential for the function of the accessory sex organs and production of the secondary sexual characteristics. They are also responsible for other effects:

Skin	● Growth of hair on chest, beard, and lower abdomen.
	● Male pattern baldness.
	● Increased sebum secretion.
Metabolic	● Anabolic effect.
	● Negative effect on gluconeogenesis.
	● Inhibitory effect on the production of lipids.
Spermatogenesis	● It seems to be accepted that androgens are indispensable for spermatogenesis, but this has not yet been fully elucidated.

The control mechanism is via the gonadotrophins through negative feed-back. There now appears to be only one release hormone (LHRH) and it seems that the changes in LH/FSH ratios are due to a modulating effect by androgens. Higher levels of androgens inhibit LH, whereas FSH may be stimulated or inhibited according to the level. Despite the long history of research on them, it is still not understood precisely how androgens work.

PATHOGENESIS OF HYPERSEXUALITY

Anatomically there is a clearly defined centre in the anterior hypothalamus, the sexual centre, which undoubtedly influences libido. This has been confirmed in patients who have grossly abnormal sexual behaviour associated with a congenital or traumatic lesion of the floor of the 3rd ventricle. The cerebral cortex obviously has a modifying influence either way, but the neurohumeral mechanism is still obscure.

The role of amines

Animal work in male and female rats has given rise to the theory that 5-hydroxytryptamine (5-HT) and dopamine have reciprocal control over sexual behaviour, 5-HT causing inhibition and dopamine causing excitation. Polypeptides have also been implicated in the pathogenesis. Nemeroff and Prange (1978) have demonstrated in ovariectomized, hypophysectomized, and adrenalectomized female rats that LHRH has a direct stimulating effect on the central nervous system (CNS) causing lordosis, a positive sign demonstrating sexual readiness.

What significance these theories have in humans is difficult to assess. The evidence to support the amine theory is weak. Laevodopa, a dopamine precursor, could be expected to cause sexual excitation, and indeed increased sexual activity has been reported in patients treated for Parkinsonism (Bowers, van Woert, and Davis 1971). This has been claimed to be unrelated to the increased neuromuscular activity (Brown, Brown, Kofman, and Quarrington 1978).

Therefore, similarly with tryptophan, a precursor of 5-HT, we should be able to predict that it has the opposite effect. Instead there have been odd reports of patients showing increased sexual activity following it's administration. In depressed patients with low levels of 5-HT, instead of sexual activity being increased, there is usually a corresponding loss of libido.

The polypeptides

Accepting that the amine theory does not answer all the clinical questions, what about the polypeptides? Again there is no real evidence for their involvement. Cyproterone acetate is an anti-gonadotrophin as well as an anti-androgen. Does it therefore exert its effect singly or in a combination of the following roles: depression of testosterone production, blockade of testosterone receptors, and depression of LHRH? If the animal data can be extrapolated to man, then an LHRH analogue should have a sexual excitatory effect. There are at least three analogues available in clinical research, but so far there is no animal or human evidence to confirm or deny this effect.

In conclusion, therefore, for the present, we have to accept that testosterone plays a role in human sexuality and that to be successful in the treatment of sexual disorders we may have to interfere with that role, understanding that in so doing we also interfere with other functions.

SEXUAL OFFENDING

Leaving the theory aside and considering the patients themselves, apart from soliciting for prostitution, sexual offending is almost exclusively a male prerogative.

Restricting the discussion to purely pharmacological methods of treatment, it can be said that since the introduction of chlorpromazine in 1954, haloperidol in 1961, and cyproterone acetate in 1974, little has changed. As far as can be seen from current research, not much is likely to change in the near future. Originally these drugs were divided arbitrarily into two groups, the non-specific and the specific.

Non-specific drugs

The non specific group appear to work through their sedative action, although they are known to affect cerebral amines and polypeptides.

The major neuroleptics, chlorpromazine, haloperidol, and in particular its close relative benperidol, seem to be the most successful and widely used. In terms of comparative efficacy, Tennent, Bancroft, and Cass (1974) demonstrated that benperidol gave superior results to chlorpromazine, particularly in measurements of frequency of sexual thoughts or sexual interest scores. The side-effects of this group of drugs can be a problem and in spite of giving orphenadrine routinely, dyskinesias are still relatively frequent. Such additional side-effects can only be a hindrance to good compliance, which is already difficult in these patients. Long-term therapy is often required and if they are in the community, rather than in prison, there are less frequent control observations.

Of the other non-specific drugs, oestrogens have been used, and Bancroft and Tennent's studies suggest that they are as effective as benperidol or the anti-androgens (Bancroft, Tennent, Loucas, and Cass 1974). However, continued use does bring the problem of gynaecomastia. Virtually all patients develop this within 2 months of commencing treatment, and there was considerable antagonism in the press a few years ago to the mastectomies that were necessary in some of these patients.

Specific measures

In the specific group, castration is of course an effective form of therapy, and has been used in Denmark with good follow-up results, but in these enlightened days 'chemical castration' with the anti-androgens is more acceptable in the UK.

Anti-androgens

A number of these compounds are now known some of which are non-steroidal such as cimetidine and flutamide, and which appear to act by inhibiting synthesis of testosterone. They are not particularly strong anti-androgens nor are they anti-gonadotrophic. Hence as they do not block the hypophyseal feedback mechanism, there may be increases in gonadotrophins and possibly also other androgens or their precursors.

The steroid compounds are more familiar. Oestrogens have already been considered. The most potent anti-androgens known at present are also progestogens: medroxyprogesterone, megestrol, chlormadinone, and cyproterone. These are all 17-hydroxy progesterone derivatives and besides exhibiting progestogenic activity, they also show weak anti-androgenic activity. Their acetates all exhibit similar strong progestogenic activity but the anti-androgenic activity is enhanced, particuarly by cyproterone acetate.

Their molecules are shown in Fig. 13.1, together with that of testosterone. Their close similarities are clear. All progestogens, including these 17-hydroxy derivatives, have been accused of causing liver tumours in rats and breast nodules in beagle dogs, at high doses. It is now accepted that the 7-year beagle dog study is not an acceptable model. The incidence of liver tumours in rats is similar with all progestogens, when comparable doses are considered, and similar to other steroids including glucocorticoids. Hence we should be reassured of their safety as far as humans are concerned.

Cyproterone acetate

Cyproterone acetate is now considered as a particular example. Its main mode of action appears to be by direct competitive blocking of androgen receptors, but it does also reduce the production of testosterone. Also, being a potent progestogen, there is an anti-gonadotrophic effect on the pituitary, and this in turn reduces the stimulus to the body to secrete endogenous testosterone. Similarly, there is a mild depressant effect on ACTH, which at least does not induce the production of other androgens or their precursor from the adrenals.

What are the clinical effects when such a compound is given? The desired effects on sexual drive, incidence of masturbation etc., have all been shown to be diminished in a number of trials, from the early ones by Laschet and Laschet

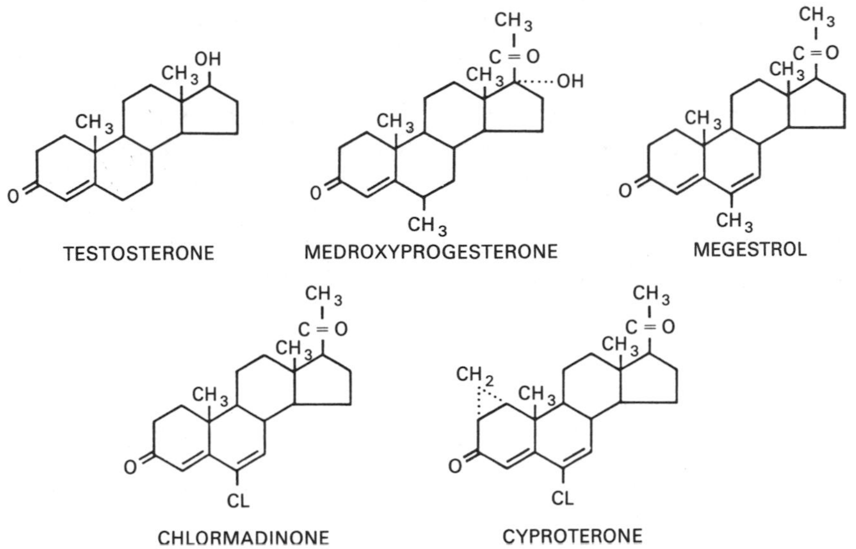

FIG. 13.1 Derivatives of 17-hydroxy progesterone with anti-androgenic activity.

(1967), to the more recent double-blind comparative studies by Tennent, Bancroft, and Cass (1974). There are of course also the undesirable effects. We are creating 'chemical eunuchs' and there are effects on skin, metabolism, and spermatogenesis, as well as on other tissues. The skin-sebum secretion rate diminishes, and there is an improvement in cases of acne. Some of the patients have reported growth of fine hair, but unfortunately the drug does not cure male-pattern baldness.

Any anti-anabolic effects seem to be transient and the effects on glucose and fat metabolism do not appear to be clinically significant. The sperm count diminishes over a period of about 6 weeks, even at doses as low as 5 mg daily. The rate of response is variable from patient to patient but, after this period of time the total count and motility are reduced to sub-fertile levels in all. After persistent treatment for 2 years or more, some patients exhibit a return to normal counts whilst continuing treatment. On stopping therapy any effects appear to be totally reversible, although in some cases it takes 6 months before the sperm count returns to normal.

With regard to undesirable effects, there is a prostogenic influence on breast tissue, and with long-term treatment, 10–15 per cent of patients are reported to develop small, firm, breast enlargements. Apart from this it does appear to be relatively free from major side-effects.

CONCLUSIONS

Current therapy appears to be limited to the sedative/depressant activity of the neuroleptics, or one or two anti-androgens. All treatments have their problems with side-effects, but they appear to be less marked with the anti-androgens.

One major problem left unsolved is compliance, particularly in out-patients.

A long-acting, injectable preparation of cyproterone acetate is available on the Continent, which could improve this, but it still cannot be obtained in this country.

Finally, what of the future? This would not appear to be in the nature of a more specific anti-androgen or even in the solution of the problems of tissue-directed drugs. I think it lies in the discovery of the pathogenesis of the condition, and it is to be hoped that the recent advances in polypeptide chemistry will contribute to this. Until this is further elucidated it appears unlikely that there will be any major contribution to the physician's therapeutic armamentarium.

References

Bancroft, J., Tennent, G., Loucas, K., and Cass, J. (1974). The control of deviant sexual behaviour by drugs: 1. Behavioural changes following oestrogens and anti-androgens. *Br. J. Psychiat.* **125**, 310–15.

Bowers, M. B., Jr., Van Woert, M., and Davis, L. (1971). Sexual behaviour during L-dopa treatment for Parkinsonism. *Am. J. Psychiat.* **127**, 1691–3.

Brown, E., Brown, G. M., Kofman, O., and Quarrington, B. (1978). Sexual function and affect in Parkinsonian men treated with L-dopa. *Am. J. Psychiat.* **135**, 1552–5.

Carney, A., Bancroft, J., and Mathews, A. (1978). Combination of hormonal and psychological treatment for female sexual unresponsiveness: a comparative study. *Br. J. Psychiat.* **132**, 339–46.

Laschet, U. and Laschet, L. (1967). Anti-androgen therapy of pathologically increased or abnormal sexuality in men. *Klin. Wochensch.* 45th year. No: 6, pp. 324–5.

Nemeroff, C. B., Prange, A. J. Jr. (1978). Peptides and psychoneuroendocrinology. A perspective. *Arch. Gen. Psychiat.* **35** (8), 999–1010.

Rada, R. T., Laws, D. R., and Kellner, R. (1976). Plasma testosterone levels in the rapist. *Psychosom. Med.* **38**, 251–68.

Tennent, G., Bancroft, J., and Cass, J. (1974). The control of deviant sexual behaviour by drugs: A double-blind, controlled study of benperidol, chlorpromazine and placebo. *Arch. Sex. Behav.* **3**, 261–71.

Vermeulen, A. and Verdonck, L. (1976). Plasma androgen levels during the menstrual cycle. *Am. J. Obstet. Gynecol.* **125**, 491–4.

Index